MOVE TO LOSE

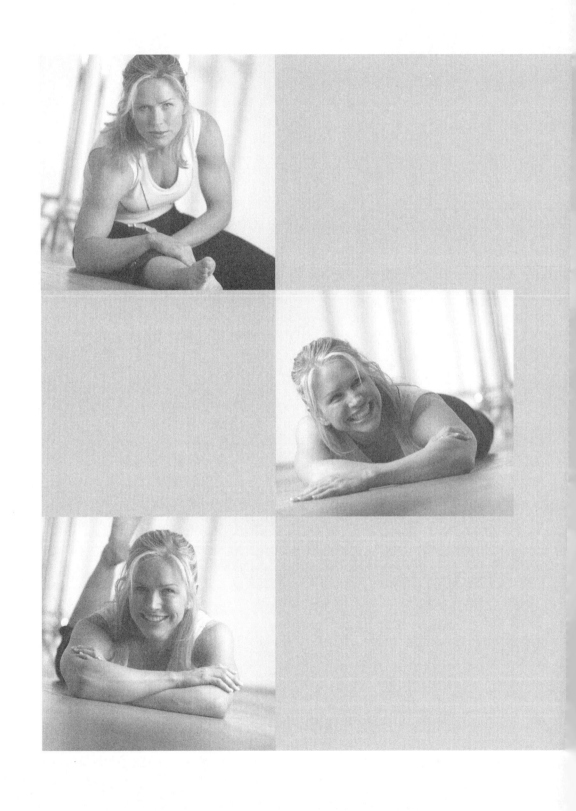

MOVE TO LOSE

Look and Feel Better in Just 10 Minutes a Day

Chris Freytag

AVERY • a member of Penguin Group (USA) Inc. • New York

AVERY

Published by the Penguin Group

Penguin Group (USA) Inc., 375 Hudson Street, New York, New York 10014, USA •
Penguin Group (Canada), 10 Alcorn Avenue, Toronto, Ontario, Canada M4V 3B2 (a division
of Pearson Penguin Canada Inc.) • Penguin Books Ltd, 80 Strand, London WC2R 0RL,
England • Penguin Ireland, 25 St Stephen's Green, Dublin 2, Ireland (a division of Penguin
Books Ltd) • Penguin Group (Australia), 250 Camberwell Road, Camberwell, Victoria 3124,
Australia (a division of Pearson Australia Group Pty Ltd) • Penguin Books India Pvt Ltd,
11 Community Centre, Panchsheel Park, New Delhi–110 017, India • Penguin Group (NZ),
Cnr Airborne and Rosedale Roads, Albany, Auckland 1310, New Zealand (a division of Pearson
New Zealand Ltd) • Penguin Books (South Africa) (Pty) Ltd, 24 Sturdee Avenue,
Rosebank, Johannesburg 2196, South Africa • Penguin Books Ltd, Registered Offices:
80 Strand, London WC2R 0RL, England

Library of Congress Cataloging-in-Publication Data

Freytag, Chris.
    Move to lose : look and feel better in just 10 minutes a day / Chris Freytag.
        p.   cm.
    Includes index.
    ISBN 1-58333-208-1
    1. Health.   2. Physical fitness.   3. Nutrition.   I. Title.

RA776.F855   2004   2004052838
613.7—dc22

Printed in the United States of America
10   9   8   7   6   5   4   3   2   1

Book design by Elizabeth Sheehan

Most Avery books are available at special quantity discounts for bulk purchase for sales promotions, premiums, fund-
raising, and educational needs. Special books or book excerpts also can be created to fit specific needs. For details,
write Penguin Group (USA) Inc. Special Markets, 375 Hudson Street, New York, NY 10014.

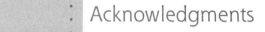

Acknowledgments

Without a doubt, this book is a labor of love for me. A huge thank-you to my husband and three children who showed love and patience through the long hours and long days. Your undying support made it possible for me to research and write this book.

Thank you to Christi Cardenas, my literary agent, whose excitement and enthusiasm were a driving force for this project. Thank you to Tom Wiese, my manager, whose continual belief in me is amazing. The two of you have been instrumental in my being able to share my message with others!

I am incredibly grateful for the time, encouragement, and wisdom Ellen Shaffer bestowed on me throughout the writing of this book. She's a gifted spirit and her influence is evident in every page.

I want to thank my clients, viewers, and family who agreed to share their stories with me and you. They are an inspiration to us all.

Dara Stewart, my editor, and her associates at Penguin Group have made this a memorable experience for me. I deeply appreciate their expertise and guidance. Thanks to Tim Pearson and Terra Hinrichs for their attention to detail and talent with the camera. Your skill helped me translate the exercises into easy-to-follow and beautiful pictures.

And a big thanks to my friends, especially Liz and Holly, who stuck by me through the process. Your unconditional support gives true meaning to the word *friend*. I must also express gratitude to my siblings and parents, who continue to be my biggest fans!

And last, but not least, thank you to everyone who has ever attended my classes, purchased my videos, or educated me in the field of health and fitness. You teachers, trainers, experts, and participants are instrumental in the journey to greater knowledge. You inspire me to motivate others!

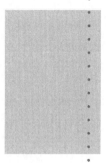

Contents

MOVE TO LOSE

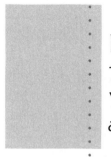

Introduction:
*Take Care of
Yourself for
a Change*

Health is not valued until sickness comes.
—DR. THOMAS FULLER

So many people need to be shocked into changing their lives for the better: a big number on the scale, a surprising test result from the doctor's office, a trip to the emergency room. But those big wake-up calls are preceded by years of smaller signals that many of us fail to hear. Maybe you're out of breath after climbing the stairs. Maybe you need a dress for a special occasion and you can't find one that fits in the size you've always worn. Maybe you're startled by how old and tired you look in the family holiday photos.

You don't have to wait for the big, scary, dramatic wake-up call. You can start waking yourself up right now.

I am certified by the American Council on Exercise (ACE) as a personal trainer, lifestyle and weight-management consultant, and a group fitness instructor. In addition to my role as the fitness expert for ShopNBC, I'm a YogaFit certified instructor and a STOTT Pilates trained instructor. Through my own business, Motivating Bodies, I've been able to work with all types of people in their homes and in corporate and health-club settings. I've spent the past fifteen years in the fitness industry and, in all that time, in my lifestyle training practice, I never met anyone who thought they had enough time to take proper care of themselves. Nobody has ever come to me because they were already eating healthy meals, getting regular exercise, drinking plenty of water, and getting enough sleep.

Like you, my clients are busy—with their jobs, their spouses, their children, their parents, and their communities. Their days are filled with meetings, errands, shopping, cooking, driving, and cleaning. They have to make sure the bills are paid, the kids have a ride to soccer practice, the family pet gets to the vet, and the dishwasher gets emptied. Caring for themselves is last on their list of priorities, if it's even on the list at all.

THE SECRET

My clients hire me hoping that I possess a secret, some kind of magic formula that will help them to change their lives. And I do have a secret. It's this:

The secret is, there is no secret.

We spend so much time, money, and energy chasing the latest diets, gimmicks, and pills. We want a painless solution that makes our body problems disappear without having to change our lives. The problem with that kind of wishful thinking is it's the way we live our lives that causes us to neglect our bodies' needs for movement, nourishment, and rest.

Realistically you're not going to eliminate the things in your life that cause you stress. You can't get rid of things like rush-hour traffic, overlapping schedules, bills to pay, kids to feed, or clothes to wash. Even though you can't eliminate stress completely, fitness fundamentals like eating well and getting regular exercise will make it much easier to manage. And you can learn coping skills, such as relaxation and meditation that will help you to put it all in perspective. Exercise can help you handle the way you perceive and handle daily stress. Then figure out how to change your perceptions and change your reactions.

I tell my clients that if they want to lose weight, they have to do it "the old-fashioned way." Just get your body moving. You need to clean up your eating. You have to eat fewer calories than you burn. And you need to fit exercise in between your family, your job, and all your other commitments.

SMALL CHANGE, BIG RESULTS

My most successful clients are realistic about who they are. They set reasonable, attainable goals. They're patient with themselves. They're not perfect all the time. They know that it's ridiculous to invest their hopes in advertising claims about quick weight loss and reshaping their bodies in thirty days. However, they get to where they want to go by making small, gradual changes that make a lasting impact on how good they look and feel. They take the ups and downs of daily life in stride and stay focused on the big picture.

I'm not reinventing the wheel. I'm going back to the basics. Life has gotten so hectic, we've forgotten about them. It's gotten too complicated. We've gotten so distracted by rigid, radical programs and none of them work.

Now that America has stopped eating carbs, you'd think we'd be able to see a difference in our nationwide waistline by now. The problem is, we are replacing calories from carbs with other processed foods and saturated fats. Look around—obesity is still an epidemic.

My program works. I've seen my clients reshape their bodies and their lives without eliminating entire food groups or exercising for two hours a day. This program is a slow, sustainable, sensible way to change your body and your mind.

Let's get started.

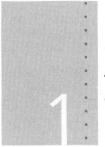

A Strong Start:
Aligning Body and Mind

We are what we repeatedly do.
—ARISTOTLE

Isn't it interesting how constant change is the driving force in our society, yet the hardest thing for us to change is ourselves? Even when we know what to do and how to do it, there's still something missing. We get sidetracked, distracted, or discouraged. Before you undertake a whole new health and fitness program, it's important to understand the connection between the body and the mind.

Every January, fitness clubs across the nation are packed with people who have the best of intentions and big plans for transforming themselves. By the end of February, almost all those newcomers are gone.

Typically something occurs after that initial motivation of starting an exercise program. If people don't see quick, visible, dramatic results, they tend to get discouraged and quit. In my years of personal training, I've seen this happen time and time again—usually at around four to six weeks.

TYPICAL PITFALLS

Here are six common mistakes that undermine most people who are just getting started—or just getting started again:

Overdoing It

If you can barely walk the next day, you sure won't be able to exercise. And if you can't exercise, you're losing a valuable chance to establish a healthy exercise habit. A little soreness and stiffness is fine; it will usually disappear once you warm up your muscles again. If the pain is sending you straight to the medicine cabinet—or right back to bed—you've pushed too hard for your current level of fitness.

Watching the Clock

There are lots of books and articles out there that tell you that you must spend at least an hour a day working out if you want to see results. If you have that kind of spare time, there's nothing wrong with this advice. But if you work full time and have kids, it's probably unrealistic. And it's discouraging—if you can't manage an hour, why bother? That's why I tell busy clients to start small. Ten minutes a day is a lot better than zero minutes a day. It'll take longer, to be sure, but it will last longer too. The key is to establish a routine that is versatile, flexible, fun, and fits your lifestyle.

Doing Too Little

If you're not breaking a sweat, breathing a bit harder, and getting your heart rate up, you're not going to see the kinds of results that will inspire you to stay with your regimen.

Checking Your Weight Every Day

Your weight can vary by several pounds daily or even within one day, depending on water and hormone fluctuations. Additionally, if you're strength training, you're building muscle, which adds weight but takes up less space than fat. So, your weight loss may not be very evident on the scale, as you may not be losing many *pounds* very quickly, but you will be losing *inches,* which is what's really important. If you're getting on the scale once a day— or more—you're setting yourself up to be discouraged. Give yourself other goals instead, like fitting into your old jeans. And if you must, weigh yourself once a week. I encourage my clients to measure their progress once a month with a tape measure instead. Measuring how many inches you've lost from your hips, waist, or thighs is a powerful motivator. Most clients tell me that fitting better in their clothes due to inches lost is often more rewarding than actual pounds lost.

Comparing Yourself to Others

Your genetics are your genetics. Your lifestyle is your lifestyle. If you won't be satisfied until you look like one of those small-boned movie stars who can afford to spend three hours every day with their private trainers, you will never think that who you are and what you can do is enough. Set your own goals and be happy in your own skin. Be proud of who you are and what you can do.

Expecting Immediate Results

We've grown accustomed to faster food, faster technology, and faster transportation, so we get impatient and disappointed when we can't take weight off as fast as we can put it on. Remember: an extra pound means you've consumed 3,500 extra calories. Get your body moving and keep it moving for a lifetime and you'll see long-term results.

THE MENTAL EDGE

Staying with a fitness program isn't always easy, especially if you are just getting started. Fitness enthusiasts, me included, will tell you that some days they've got it—and some days they don't.

I believe that 50 percent of staying with your program is mental! The only difference between you and all those regular exercisers out there is that they stick with their plan. They've mastered the mental edge.

When you see someone who is physically fit, they seem more energetic. They have a glow and a visible zest for life. Their relationships and actions seem more solid. They have discovered that

Perspectives from My Client Files

Angie E. is a busy mom who has been my client for three years. She listened, she followed my advice, and she was patient. Most of all, she worked hard and remained realistic.

She started eating smaller, healthier portions but she didn't deprive herself. She worked hard at exercise, honoring her commitment to five or six days a week.

When Angie has a crazy day, or misses a workout, she doesn't give up. She just gets right back into her groove.

"It's finally just part of my lifestyle," she told me one day. "I wake up and plan where and how to get my workout in. It's not a question of whether I will do it. It's part of my routine—like brushing my teeth!"

Angie lost thirty pounds and two or three dress sizes before her most recent pregnancy. At press time, she was almost back down to her pre-pregnancy weight.

the way they feel is far more satisfying than eating junk and being sedentary ever was. That's the mental edge!

So how do you stay committed? Few people are actually born desiring to get up at 5:00 A.M. to do a workout. But I know from personal experience that it's a behavior that can be learned because the rewards are so great. It took me a good six months until I could honestly say that I became addicted to morning exercise. Now, if I skip my morning workout, the consequences are so great that I'm conditioned to get up just to avoid the bad feeling and to experience the endorphin rush I've become addicted to.

As Aristotle said, "We are what we repeatedly do." So the mental edge isn't something you can acquire before you get started. It's something that grows inside you and gets a little bit stronger with every healthy decision you make. To free your mind, move your body.

Exercise can be like falling in love. At first it seems exciting, and then the novelty wears off. There will be lots of times when you'll want to revert back to your old, unhealthy ways. Remember, giving up is a conscious choice—and you don't have to make it. You need to tap into the strongest, most committed parts of yourself. You need to make a promise to yourself and honor it just as much as you honor the promises you make to others. That's what I mean by commitment.

You need to explore new exercises when your workouts get stale. You need to forgive yourself when you get off track and return to your healthy new habits as quickly as you can. It only takes one workout to get back in the game.

Most of all, you need to understand that it takes plenty of patience and plenty of time to make lasting, healthy changes in your body composition; there is no quick fix. Even the smallest of lifestyle changes will have a powerful effect over time. Regular exercise and sensible eating is the only way to achieve lasting results.

Or look at it this way: Whether you think you can or you think you can't, you're right!

MOTIVATION MATTERS

I know it isn't easy. I'm asking you to make a huge change—and not only in the way you eat and exercise. I'm asking you to live your life and forget your age. You don't have to settle for a slowing metabolism, diminishing muscle tone, fragile bones, and ever-diminishing energy. I'm asking you to work within your framework. And I understand that changing your life so dramatically can seem completely unattainable and unrealistic some days. But I also know that you have so much to gain. The time you invest in movement, good nutrition, proper hydration, and adequate rest will pay you back a hundred times over by giving you more energy to do the working, commuting, parenting, cooking, and cleaning. And you'll have enough energy left over to have a little fun!

Movement is one of the best solutions to your personal energy crisis. It makes you feel good about yourself, which makes you more productive. It won't make your stress go away. But it will make it so much easier to manage.

Gaining energy and managing stress aren't the only benefits that make a healthy lifestyle so worthwhile. If you're a parent, you'll be improving the example you're setting for your children and increasing their odds of leading a longer, happier, healthier life. Those of us who are parents are blessed with one of the best motivators in the world. If you won't do it for yourself, I urge you to do it for your kids.

A child born in 2000 has a one-in-three chance of developing type 2 diabetes. And a 2003 study by researchers in the United States, Australia, and Sweden showed that American children are the heaviest, least active children in the world. Kids are sponges. So set an example.

Many of us find it hard to spend money on ourselves. But we find it easy to spend it on our kids. If this sounds like you, try thinking about every dollar and every minute you spend on yourself as if you were spending them on your children. If you give yourself what you need, you'll have the physical and mental energy you need to give them what they need too.

If you still find yourself in need of motivation, think about your old age. I tell my clients we're all in training for our senior years. Someone at the gym asked me, "Hey, what are you training for?" I said, "I'm training for life!" Today's good habits will pay off tomorrow, giving you the flexibility to reach up into your cupboards, the strength to carry your own groceries, and the endurance you'll need to play with your grandkids. Keep up the good work and you'll keep yourself out of assisted living. My late grandma Eileen, who died at eighty-four, was full of energy, a real talker, and a true believer in the power of positive affirmations. My other grandmother, Doris, is still totally independent at ninety-one.

When it comes to motivation, one size never fits all. What motivates each of us depends on our individual lives and circumstances. So I encourage my clients to spend some time with a journal, thinking and writing about why they want to change their bodies.

Almost all motivation is good motivation. But the motivation of vanity can be a little tricky. Of course we are all vain to some degree. Just don't let it be your primary motivator. Vanity may feel like a very powerful impetus at first, especially if you're trying to drop a dress size or two before a class reunion or a big wedding coming up in three weeks. But if you take care of yourself, your energy, your needs, and your vanity will be satisfied. You'll have a glow. You'll look better. And the long run is what I want you to be thinking about. So balance your vanity with a measure of concern for your health and well-being. The pursuit of health and fitness is a journey, not a destination. So go with the changes in your life, age, and body and continue to feed the fountain of longevity.

THE DOWNSIDE OF DISCIPLINE

Another pitfall that might seem like a good idea is starting a big, overwhelming program of extreme diet and exercise. Going overboard with severely restricted eating and/or strenuous exercise is really just as bad as overeating and getting no exercise at all. Often, people who want to change their bodies for the better will try to make up for months or years of unhealthy living with a few short weeks of strict dieting and punishing workouts.

Perhaps you've tried this approach. At first, everything seems to go fine. You clear your kitchen of bread, carrots, fruit, or whatever else the celebrity diet of the minute forbids you to eat. Or you set your alarm for four-thirty in the morning five days a week so you can run five miles and do fifty sit-ups before the kids wake up. I see a lot of this every January, as people are making their New Year's resolutions.

At first, your new regimen might feel like it's going pretty well. You probably see a few pounds disappear. You feel disciplined and in control. But sooner or later, you get tired of all that huffing and puffing. Your knees start to ache and you "accidentally" oversleep. Or you'll be invited out to a restaurant and find yourself being overpowered by the aromas wafting from the breadbasket.

So you'll eat the bread or skip the run and feel like a failure. You'll get discouraged and depressed. You'll console yourself with comfort food and feel even worse.

If this sounds like something you've experienced, let me reassure you that you're not alone. Dieting without exercise has a 95 percent failure rate. Ninety-five percent of those who lose weight gain it back with a little extra padding!

Actually, all your previous attempts to lose weight and get in shape have not been failures. They've been lessons—valuable lessons your body has been teaching you about how it works. Fortunately, putting those lessons into practice isn't rocket science. It's just a matter of taking the information I'm going to give you and finally having a doable, organized plan to sustain a lifestyle change.

BODY BASICS

Once you understand how your metabolism works, you'll never want to go on a deprivation diet again. Our bodies are designed to store fat so that we can survive famine. This kept our ancestors alive despite natural disasters like droughts and floods that would wipe out their food supply. When our ancestors couldn't get enough to eat, their metabolism would slow down so that they'd burn fewer calories. Once the food supply resumed, they replenished their fat stores so they could live long enough to pass along this slow-burning, fat-hoarding genetic heritage to us.

To your body, a calorie-restricted diet feels just like a famine. Your metabolism has no idea that you can, in fact, get to a well-stocked supermarket in a matter of minutes. So your metabolic rate slows down. You burn fewer calories. And you hit a plateau, no longer losing any weight, even though you're hungry all the time.

So breaking your diet doesn't mean you're weak or undisciplined.

In Her Own Words and Pictures

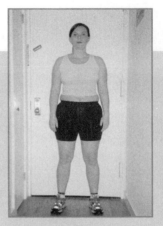

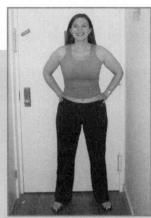

1.1 • Katie (before)   1.2 • Katie (after)

My sister, Katie, pictured at right, lost fifteen pounds in sixty days—and she's still losing. This is her story:

Growing up I was always active, playing sports through high school and remaining athletic through college. It was during the post-college years that I began to lose my figure. I worked all the time and was very social. I went out to dinner and happy hours with friends. I quickly lost my motivation to go to the gym. Within two years I had gained thirty pounds, and no matter what I tried for the next several years, I could not seem to take the weight off. I would lose five pounds and then gain ten.

Every time I came to see you, you would try to motivate me to get back into shape. You would keep telling me to "eat clean" and get my butt to the gym. Of course, that was not what I wanted to hear. So I kept trying every gimmick—I wouldn't eat carbs; or I'd eat specific percentages of carbs, protein, and fat; or I wouldn't eat sugar; or I'd fast on fruit juice for twenty days. These were completely unrealistic for someone like me, who lives in New York City, doesn't cook, and is social.

You kept telling me, "It is a simple formula, Katie, calories in versus calories out." So I just ate in moderation and I finally started to go to the gym. I found some aerobic classes that motivated me to go. I went and exercised when *Oprah* was on so that I was motivated. I incorporated the gym into my schedule, and now it is habit.

All my friends keep asking me how I lost fifteen pounds without starving myself or restricting myself. They noticed my attitude seemed to be more positive than in the past about working out. First of all, I have found that the more consistently I work out, the more consistent my good mood is. I feel like working out now is like a happy drug. It makes my body and attitude feel better. As far as the eating, I have stopped eating processed foods and foods that are not "clean." I started eating egg substitutes like Egg Beaters and whole-wheat toast in the morning instead of a bagel or muffin. I started eating more vegetables. I started backing off the pasta, rice, and white breads. The trick is that I did not do this all at once but gradually. When I go out to eat, I ask for more vegetables instead of potatoes. I am no longer afraid of eating healthy fats found in nuts and avocados. Actually, they make me feel full. I eat what I want in moderation.

The other key is that it has to be a lifestyle change, not a quick fix. I needed to sit down and figure out how to change my life, how to incorporate fitness into my daily schedule, and how to pick healthy choices when eating out. Finally, I realized that I needed to get control of my health and make a plan.

I am only young once and I don't want to be overweight for the entire time.

And hitting a plateau doesn't mean you should starve yourself to get your weight-loss momentum going again. It just means that you can only defy your genes for so long.

This metabolic slowdown is the reason why so many dieters eventually regain all the weight they lose. If, for example, you were burning 2,000 calories a day before you started your diet, you might be burning only 1,800 calories a day after a few weeks of dieting. When you resume eating normally, you'll actually gain weight faster because your body thinks it needs to conserve energy. It's the opposite of being a well-fueled engine, consuming enough fuel so your body continues to burn calories.

At this point, losing weight might seem just about impossible. Your busy life is working against you. Your metabolism is working against you. But knowledge is power, and knowing just how much you're up against will help you get to where you want to be. You can do it. I've seen plenty of success stories in my career as a lifestyle trainer.

SET YOUR GOALS AND MAKE SOME PLANS

Having a vague idea that you "should" get some more exercise and rethink your eating probably hasn't worked for you in the past. So don't make that mistake again.

Grab a fresh, new notebook or sit down at your computer and open a new document. Your first assignment is to identify a long-term goal.

Ask yourself what you want to accomplish. And write down your answers. Be as specific as you can. Here are some examples of long-term goals:

- I want to lose fifteen pounds in the next six months.
- I want to lower my blood pressure by ten points.

Ten Minutes to Tranquility

If you've been looking for a way to solve your daily stress, look no further than your own mind. Meditation is a vital part of healthy living. It's your time to devote to your inner fitness. Doctors are starting to recommend meditation as a way to improve your health. Meditation can be spiritual or religious, depending on how you want to think about it. But at the simplest, most fundamental level, meditation is just facilitated self-reflection. It's a time to clear your head, take in some oxygen, and set aside any outside distractions.

Set a kitchen timer for ten minutes. Then sit down, get comfortable, and meditate. The simplest form of meditation is to just focus on your breathing. Just pay attention to how your chest expands and contracts, how your lungs and rib cage rise and fall like a balloon. When thoughts occur to you, just mentally set them aside and return your focus on your breathing. Whenever your mind strays, just gently bring your awareness back to the rhythm of your breath.

We take approximately 21,000 breaths a day. Breathing is movement at its most basic level—a form of exercise. It burns calories and increases circulation.

- I want to participate in a 5K walk/run next Memorial Day.
- I want to be two dress sizes smaller by my fortieth birthday.

Notice how all those goals begin with "I want." Your long-term goal should really feel like it belongs to you, like it's right for your body and appropriate for your lifestyle. If you're trying to lose weight because your spouse wants you to, or even if your doctor recommends it, it won't have the same psychological power as a goal you really want for yourself.

Once you declare your long-term goal, the next step is to break your goal down into short-term goals. Be fair and kind to yourself: Be realistic about how much time it will take to achieve exactly what you want. Examples of short-term goals include:

- I will start by getting ten minutes of exercise a day for the first two weeks; then I will find another five minutes for a total of fifteen minutes a day.
- I will add up how many calories I consume in a typical day and identify ways I can cut out 500 per day.
- I will buy a balance ball and do ten minutes of core-strengthening exercises four days a week for a month.

Here are some goal-setting guidelines to follow:

- *A plan is imperative.* To lose a pound a week, you need to create a deficit of about 500 calories per day between diet and exercise. One way is to split those 500 calories equally between diet and exercise. Find a way to move your body and burn 250 more calories. Find a way to eat 250 fewer calories.
- *Set reachable and realistic goals.* Don't set a goal that is completely unattainable, like returning to how much you weighed when you were twenty. Be realistic about who you are today.
- *Reward yourself for little successes.* If your long-term goal is to lose a total of fifty pounds, that's going to take some time. Focus instead on having a good day or a good week. Over time, those good days and good weeks will add up to a healthy, new lifestyle. Choose rewards that support your healthy lifestyle changes. Treat yourself to some cute new workout clothes or a subscription to a health and

fitness magazine. Rewards don't always have to mean spending money. If you stick to your plan to exercise five days in one week, reward yourself on Friday with a thirty-minute bubble bath.

- *Be flexible.* You will almost certainly have ups and downs. Nobody's perfect—even the most dedicated exercisers get stuck in traffic and come down with the flu sometimes. Some days will be harder than others. Some days will unravel despite the best of plans. Don't give up. Just get back on track the next day.

Once you've identified your goals, don't put away your notebook. Your next task is to figure out how to get there. It's time to create a plan.

If your short-term goal calls for exercising ten minutes a day, what's the best time in the day for you to find those ten minutes? Where's the best place? If you're a morning person, maybe you can set your alarm clock fifteen minutes earlier. If you're absolutely not a morning person, maybe you can exercise in the evening, when you're normally watching television. Your body knows no difference; you burn the same number of calories whether you're watching Katie Couric or Jay Leno.

If your workplace is close to a fitness club or a walking path, maybe you can exercise duirng your lunch hour. If the nearest gym is across town, you might be more likely to succeed if you plan to do most of your workouts at home.

If your goals include cutting calories, how will you do that? You'll probably feel less deprived if you cut some calories by making substitutions instead of declaring, "No cookies again, ever!" Try replacing the 2-percent milk in your morning latte with skim, and replace the whipped cream with a sugar-free flavor shot or a dusting of cinnamon. Replace your potato chips with air-popped popcorn? If plain popcorn doesn't appeal to you, spritz it with a little olive oil and sprinkle it with a little seasoning salt. There are any number of small changes you can make in your diet that can lead to big rewards.

If these decisions are hard to make, try keeping a food diary for a

---

Top Ten Ways to Make the Most of Ten Minutes

Here's a small change to get you started: Be kind to yourself for ten minutes. Ten minutes is enough to:

- Make yourself a cup of green tea.
- Drink a tall glass of water.
- Make a healthy grocery list.
- Prepare a healthy meal or snack.
- Take a walk, just around the block.
- Stretch your body.
- Meditate.
- Write in your journal.
- Do some strength training on an exercise ball while watching TV or playing with your kids.
- Shop online for a beginner's workout on video or DVD—something you've always wanted to try, like yoga or Pilates.

week. Write down everything you eat, what time you eat it, and how hungry you were. Notice when you tend to overeat. Some people are afternoon snackers. Some nosh in the evenings after dinner. You might notice you eat more at social gatherings or at home in front of the television. I've noticed that I tend to snack and sample while I'm fixing dinner. Now I chew sugarless bubble gum or pull out a bag of baby carrots to keep my jaw moving. And I used to clear my kids' plates by eating their leftovers rather than putting them in the garbage. Those extra calories never registered in my mind. My generation was raised to feel guilty about wasting food. But I realized that eating the crusts from my kids' sandwiches didn't do a thing to help world hunger.

Here are some keys to successful planning:

- Sweat the details. Figure out where you're going to exercise—and when. Figure out what you're going to eat and when.

- Don't carve your plan in stone. Plan your week to the best of your ability. Try to anticipate anything that might throw you for a loop, like a family birthday party or a difficult deadline. It's always easier to come up with a Plan B before you really need one. If you're consistently having a hard time sticking to your plan, don't beat yourself up. Just change your plan. Educate yourself. What you don't know can hurt you. Knowledge is power. The more you learn about your body and nutrition, the easier it will be for you to stick to your program.

- Start small. Begin by committing to move your body at least three days a week. As your fitness improves and your energy increases, change your routine to four days a week. Then work toward five.

- Pace yourself. This is vital if you're doing strength training. Your body needs a rest if you are sore so that the muscles can rest and rebuild. Start with two days a week; once you're stronger, you can make it three days a week.

- Make room for variety. Our bodies get bored eating the same foods over and over. The same goes for exercise. Changing your workout periodically will help you avoid plateaus and keep your

Numbers That Count

0 is the number of cigarettes you should smoke. After your first smoke-free year, you cut your risk for heart disease in half!

1/2 gram per pound of body weight per day is how much protein you should be eating if you are moderately to very physically active. For example, a 130-pound woman should aim to eat 65 grams of protein daily.

6 mini meals per day is a great way to stay fueled, maintain portion control, and keep your body running efficiently.

10 minutes is all you need to benefit from a workout if you are just getting started. Every little effort counts. When you're just beginning, consistency is more important than intensity.

30 minutes of daily exercise puts you in line with the most recent government recommendations to help reduce your risk for many diseases.

60 days is how long it takes to form a habit. Move your body for 60 days in a row and you're on your way to a permanent lifestyle change!

120/80 or below is considered normal healthy blood pressure. Check your blood pressure regularly. Maintain healthy blood pressure by eating foods rich in calcium, potassium, and magnesium.

200 is the upper limit for total cholesterol. 130–160 for LDL is borderline high. 160 and above is the upper limit for LDL (bad) cholesterol. Ideally, your LDL cholesterol count should be less than 100. Your HDL (good) cholesterol count should be 40 or higher. To keep your cholesterol at a healthy level, exercise and increase your intake of fruits and vegetables.

3,500 is the number of calories in one pound. Losing one pound means creating a deficit of 3,500 calories. This cannot be done in a day, no matter what the advertisements for crash diets imply. Do it gradually and you're doing it right: Cut back 500 calories a day for one week to lose a pound.

21,000 breaths a day. That's approximately how many breaths it takes to sustain life.

mind engaged in what your body is doing. Why not try a new fruit or a new fitness class once a month? If you've never tasted a mango or participated in a kickboxing class, see what you're missing!

- Start at your level. If you haven't exercised in several years, you're not going to be happy in an intermediate Spinning class. The biggest mistake beginners make is taking on too much too soon. That can lead to injury, burnout, and discouragement. Start with baby steps. Every journey begins with that first step.

Finally, don't give in to the temptation to skip the goal-setting and planning process. If you were driving somewhere you'd never been before, would you just jump in the car and go without getting directions? Would you expect to find your way just because you wanted to get there? Of course not! If you're changing your life, you're going somewhere you've never been before. So setting your goals and making your plans is like reading a map and getting directions. If you do this, you can succeed.

Keep reading!

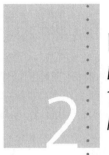

Losing to Win:
Ditching the Myths
That Don't
Measure Up

To remain young one must change.
—ALEXANDER CHASE

Before we start to work on your hips, we need to work on your head. If you're not happy with your body, you probably have a lot to lose—and I don't mean pounds. I mean misconceptions, excuses, and bad habits.

Your body didn't come with an owner's manual. And, unless you majored in physiology, you were probably never taught much about what your body needs and how it works. Most of us learn about eating and exercise haphazardly from advertisements, television shows, magazines, and media sponsored by businesses that are marketing their products to us.

In my practice, I see so many bright, educated, and successful people who are trying to operate their bodies with information that's incomplete, out of date, or just plain wrong. So let's warm up by shedding a few half-truths.

LOSE YOUR MISCONCEPTIONS

Misconception #1: Strength Training Isn't for Me

Starting in our thirties, we lose one-half to one pound of muscle a year. This affects more than our ability to haul groceries from the car to the kitchen. Muscle is your body's calorie-burning furnace. If you let your muscle mass diminish without cutting calories, middle-aged weight gain is inevitable. But cutting calories isn't the only way to cope.

One of the best things you can do to boost your calorie-burning rate is to build muscle. The more muscle you have, the more calories your body needs, even at rest. This is why men can eat so much more than women without gaining weight—the typical man is built with more muscle than the typical woman.

Strength training to build muscle is one of the most important things you can do to manage your weight. Not only does it help you to burn more calories, muscle helps you look better: A pound of muscle takes up about 18 percent less space than a pound of fat.

Many women avoid strength training because they don't want to look bulky or masculine. But the body of a competitive female body-builder requires many, many hours of lifting very heavy weights to counter-act the bulk-preventing effects of estrogen. That kind of highly developed musculature never ever happens by accident. The regimen I recommend uses lighter weights and more reps to sculpt lean muscle mass.

Many women prefer cardio to strength training because they're focused on burning calories. But cardio alone won't sculpt your muscles. To do that, you need to exercise with weights or resistance.

Misconception #2: Carbohydrates Are Bad
The current popularity of high-protein diets has caused many people to conclude that eating carbohydrate-rich foods like bread, fruit, and starchy vegetables makes you fat. Although it's true that *over*eating these foods will make you gain weight, overeating any food group will make you gain weight. Carbs themselves are not evil. They are an essential nutrient, the most easily accessible energy source your body has at its disposal. Without energy, your body simply can't function properly.

All carbohydrate-rich foods are not created equal, however. Fiber-rich, minimally processed grains, fruits, and vegetables will give you more nourishment, and a more satisfying sense of fullness, than breads made from refined, chemically bleached flour or crackers made with unhealthy fats. See chapter 4 for more information about the role of carbohydrates in a healthy program of clean eating.

Misconception #3: Fat Is Bad

Diet fads change like hemline fashions; before low-carb diets were in vogue, low-fat diets were thought to be the be-all and end-all of weight control. Many of the "fat-free" foods you see on the supermarket shelves today are the result of the fat-free diet fads of the 1980s. And consumers routinely gobble up entire bags of fat-free treats like cookies, thinking that they're getting away with something that won't show up on the scale later. But fat-free isn't calorie-free; in fact, manufacturers compensate for the absence of fat in many fat-free foods by adding more sugar to their recipes. Even with the extra sugar, most of these products don't taste as good as the foods they imitate. Fats provide flavorful and satisfying qualities to foods like cookies, salad dressings, and cheeses.

Fat, despite its bad reputation, is actually a necessary nutrient. Deprive yourself of fat and you'll be depriving yourself of smooth skin and shiny hair. You'll also deprive your system of essential, fat-soluble vitamins, like vitamin E. And scientists have recently discovered that your body needs fat to burn fat. A fat-free diet can actually prevent you from losing excess weight!

Fat got its bad name because it's high in calories. And there are some fats, such as saturated animal fats and the chemically altered trans fats (also known as "partially hydrogenated oils"), used in many prepared and processed foods, that you're better off avoiding whenever possible. But there are plenty of healthy fat-rich foods—such as olive oil, tuna, and nuts—that can actually make weight control easier. See chapter 4 for specifics.

LOSE YOUR EXCUSES

Excuse #1: *I'm Too Overweight to Exercise*

Some people are afraid to join a gym because they think they'll be the only overweight person there. I've been teaching group fitness classes at health clubs for years, and I can tell you that you will always find people of all shapes, sizes, and ages. And most gym goers will be far too focused on their own bodies to pay any attention to yours. Recently, the industry has seen a whole new phenomenon: fitness clubs that offer thirty-minute workouts in a supportive, easy-to-navigate environment. Workout facilities such as

Curves are designed especially to make women feel comfortable as they get started with exercise.

Even if a gym is just not right for you, you have plenty of other options. Put on a pair of walking shoes and start striding through your neighborhood in the morning. If you simply can't bear the thought of exercising in public, you can exercise in the privacy of your own home with just a few pieces of equipment and some great music to get your heart going. See chapter 6, "Moving Parts," for advice on setting up your very own home gym. You'll be amazed with what you can do without a lot of space or a ton of cash.

If you're concerned that you will injure or overexert yourself, I encourage you to make an appointment with your doctor. He or she can help you determine what's right and what's risky for your present age, weight, and fitness level. Whatever your current fitness level, start with baby steps. You're never too old. And it's never too late. Whether you start sitting or standing, it's got to happen! It's not what you do today. It's what you do this week, this month, this year!

Excuse #2: *I Don't Have Time for Healthy Meals*
You don't have time to wash an apple? Of course you do! In the time it takes you to microwave something that comes in a box, you can rinse some salad greens, add some cooked chicken, slice a tomato, and sprinkle some chopped walnuts. The catch is: You have to have the ingredients in your kitchen and ready to go. And that takes planning. If there's nothing in your fridge but old produce and even older condiments, there's nothing to keep you from ordering something supersized from the drive-thru. We'll talk more about meal planning in chapter 4. There's no valid excuse for poor nutrition in our society, where choice is so abundant.

Excuse #3: *Exercise Is Boring*
If by "exercise" you mean trudging on a treadmill day in and day out with nothing to think about but how much time you have left before you can stop, then you're absolutely right. It is boring. But it doesn't have to be. Variety is essential to healthy movement. So is playfulness.

When you were a kid, exercise was fun because you didn't call it exercise. You called it "riding bikes" or "going swimming" or "playing tag."

At what age did we stop having fun through movement? Where is it written that, at some point, we're too old to ride bikes? Laughter is great exercise—it uses the muscles in your face, your shoulders, your chest, and even your abdominals. Six-year-olds laugh hundreds of times a day. Grownups are lucky if they can squeeze in ten.

As adults, we think of exercise as a chore, as just one more item on our endless list of things we're supposed to do. So try putting activities like these on your list: Play hide-and-seek with your kids, play Frisbee with your dog, or play tennis with your spouse on Saturday mornings. The important word here is "play." If you have to go indoors, make your treadmill fun. Read or watch a movie while walking or running. Or listen to great music.

My clients always ask me what kind of exercise burns the most calories. My answer is always the same: It's the exercise you like the best. If you like it, you'll keep doing it. And that's how you burn the most calories.

Excuse #4: *I Don't Have Time to Exercise*

I know you're busy. And I know it's hard. I know because I have three kids and a career. I've seen people try to lose weight with an obsessive, crazy workout schedule only to be so sore and tired, they're incapable of doing it again the next day. That's why I've created the moderate, time-efficient workouts you'll find in chapters 7 through 10. Let's work on maximum results in minimum time.

The calories you burn at 6 P.M. are no better or no worse than the calories you burn at 6 A.M. The important thing is to work on your cumulative caloric burn throughout the day. A ten-minute workout is a great way to start the day, first thing in the morning before anyone else in the house is awake. If you are really, truly not a morning person, try fitting ten minutes of exercise into your lunch break. Or do it first thing in the evening, as soon as you get home, while you're watching your favorite news show or sitcom. If you manage to do all three, congratulations! Those thirty minutes of exercise are just as good for you as one single thirty-minute session.

Of course there are going to be days when you truly can't find even ten minutes because you have a sick toddler or a big presentation due or a plumbing emergency. That's okay. The road to good health is always under

Top Reasons to Ditch the Diet Cycle Forever! 10

1. *Diets are disastrous.* The problem with diets is plain and simple, they do not work! They are too restrictive, too sudden, and too unrealistic. Diets are created by people who know nothing about your taste buds, lifestyle, emotions, and hormones, not to mention what your family will or won't tolerate at the dinner table. Let's face it, most diets are impossible to follow for a lifetime. Focus instead on making gradual, healthy changes to your eating habits.

2. *Diets are short-term.* The quick-fix approach has proven ineffective—both in the labs and in real life. Once you succumb to temptation or go back to living a normal lifestyle, you are no better off than before you started dieting.

3. *Diets are trendy.* We've tried them all: There was the grapefruit diet, the cabbage-soup diet, and too many others that have done absolutely nothing to make a dent in the rising rates of obesity. These diets are restrictive, unscientific, and gimmicky. They don't last a lifetime. Most people can only stay with them for a few weeks to a month—which is about how long it takes for any weight they lose to come right back.

4. *Diets cause depletion.* It's no coincidence that the first three letters of "diet" spell "die," because that's exactly what happens to your energy level. Drastically reducing your calorie intake and eliminating certain nutrients from your body can cause your moods to change. Dieting leaves you feeling tired, lethargic, and irritable. You can't think clearly about anything except your next meal. Your body needs fuel to function properly. If you're consuming too little, your metabolism will shift into starvation mode and your body will hold onto every fat cell. By slowing down the rate at which your body burns calories, dieting can actually cause those frustrating plateaus, where the scale won't budge, even though you're eating like a bird. To keep your energy high and your metabolism running smoothly, keep your body fueled with five or six mini-meals per day.

5. *Diets cause deficiencies.* Any diet that eliminates an entire food group isn't going to be healthy and provide you with the balanced nutrients you need every day. Being overweight is enough of a health problem; don't make matters even worse by risking vitamin and mineral deficiencies.

6. *Diets are too rigid.* Diets often require extra effort and time for calorie counting, measuring, and concocting strange recipes. Diets usually aren't adaptable for the whole family, so you have to buy additional foods and become a short-order cook.

7. *Diets create low self-esteem.* With so many restrictions and rules, you are almost guaranteed to fail. Drastic changes in eating habits lead to quitting. Small, gradual changes make it easier to succeed over the long haul.

8. *Diets can be costly!* Diet programs often require special pre-packaged meals and snacks. Keeping your kitchen stocked with these special foods is almost always expensive and almost never convenient.

9. *Diets are all-consuming.* The more you diet, the more food-obsessed you get. Eat to live; don't live to eat!

10. *Diets have no guarantees.* Making small lifestyle and behavior changes is what leads to real weight loss for the long term. It takes time to put the weight on; it takes even more time to take the weight off. A quick fix will never change who you are deep down. Only gradual habit and lifestyle changes will make a lasting impact!

construction. Once in a while, you're going to have to stop and park. Just don't stay there. Make sure you find the time the next day.

Excuse #5: *It's My Genetics*

This is true to a point: Genetics play a role in cholesterol levels and heart disease. But 70 percent of aging is lifestyle. So the choices you make every day are just as important—perhaps more important—in determining how long you live and how well you feel.

LOSE YOUR BAD HABITS

Bad Habit #1: *All-or-Nothing Thinking*

So many people think they have to be strict with themselves, insisting on perfection, accepting nothing less than 100 percent: If you're not totally good at sticking to your diet and exercise regimen, then you're bad; if you're not a success, you're a failure; if you're not as thin as you want to be, you must be fat.

This kind of thinking will sabotage you eventually because you're going to cheat, slip, and fail every once in a while. Everyone does. It's human. And it's okay to indulge—even a couple of times a week.

Recently a woman e-mailed me to ask what I thought about the idea of "free days," where you allocate one day a week to eat anything you want. I don't believe the free day is a good idea. It's too rigid. If you're going out to dinner with friends and everybody's splitting dessert, what are you going to do if it isn't your free day? And I don't think it's smart to encourage anyone to eat junk food just because it's a particular day. I advise my clients to live a normal life. If a glass of wine would be great on Tuesday, don't save it until Saturday.

No one wants to feel deprived. Living without ever enjoying birthday cake, chocolate, and your grandmother's recipe for turkey stuffing isn't really living. But living on nothing but cake, chocolate, and stuffing isn't living well.

Aim instead for a happy medium, with realistic goals. Life is not perfect. If you think otherwise, you set yourself up for failure. You've got to have options, plans, and backup plans. Treat yourself *just* often enough so it really feels like a treat. It's not just a matter of willpower for a short period of time; it's a lifestyle change, a new way of thinking. I'm going to show you how to set expectations that realistically fit your lifestyle, keep your goals attainable, and question those aspirations that don't really work to your benefit. (You want to reach your high-school weight . . . why?)

Bad Habit #2: *Supersized Portions*

In the 1950s, a single-serving bottle of cola was six ounces and contained about 80 calories. Today it's hard to find any bottles smaller than sixteen or twenty ounces. Soft drink cups from convenience stores and fast-food places can weigh in at sixty-four ounces, which comes to about 800 calories! Even a regular can of cola contains a quarter cup of white sugar. A serving of pasta, according to the nutritional information on the side of the package, weighs two ounces before cooking. At your favorite Italian restaurant, the serving on your plate is probably three times that size. A serving of meat is three ounces, about the size of the palm of your hand or a pack of playing cards. But you'd never know it from looking at the menu at a typical steak place, where the smallest sirloin on the menu is at least twice that big. Bakery cookies, once bite-sized, now resemble Frisbees.

You'll find oversized portions everywhere, even in foods that you're sure are good for you. The message behind the marketing of food tells you that bigger sizes mean better value, encouraging you to eat more. If you're in the habit of picking up a bottled fruit smoothie to go with your lunch, check out the nutrition label on the side. Look for "number of servings per container." If it's a sixteen-ounce bottle, it probably contains two servings. So if the label says it contains 200 calories per serving, and you drink the whole bottle, you're drinking an extra 400 calories with your lunch.

When we were kids, our mothers trained us to clean our plates. As adults we have to train ourselves to do the opposite. When you order an entrée in a restaurant, ask your waiter to bring you a take-home container along with your meal. Then put half of it into the container before you take a single bite. Out of sight means out of mind.

Portion control is a problem for adults but it's an even bigger problem for kids. We are setting kids up for trouble by insisting that they belong to the clean-plate club. Portions were smaller back then. Even dinner plates were 20 percent smaller than they are now! I'm always seeing parents plopping adult-sized portions on kids' plates. Remember, smaller bodies need smaller portions.

See chapter 4 for more helpful hints on portion control.

Bad Habit #3: *Skipping Meals*

Whenever you skip a meal, you force your body to operate with low blood sugar. Having low blood sugar depletes your energy, ruins your mood, impairs your judgment, and leaves you vulnerable to temptations like vending machine candy bars, entire bags of potato chips, gigantic restaurant portions, and other high-calorie disasters that will more than make up for the 400 calories you thought you were saving by skipping breakfast.

Sensible Plan, Sensational Results

It is so great to have people recognize the progress I have made. People always ask how I lost thirty pounds and went from a 36 waist to a 32. My response: "Commitment!" For years, I made statements like "I need to lose weight," or "I'm so out of shape." But nothing ever happened because I was not committed.

Then, for the first time, I really decided to commit myself to losing weight and getting in shape. I told myself "I'm going to lose twenty pounds." I made a commitment to eat only what was good for me, to cut back on portion size, and to exercise at least three times a week. For six months, I avoided fried foods, chocolate, and fattening spreads. I ate until I was content, rather than stuffed. When entertaining clients or friends, I had one glass of red wine instead of a couple of pints of beer. If I missed a workout, I made it up later in the week. Exercise became a part of my life and I never ended a week without three workouts. Chris, you've been telling me this for years. And I finally did it.

Within three months, I lost twenty pounds easily. Because I changed my lifestyle, I lost another ten pounds. I have kept the weight off for more than a year. Sure, I have a piece of chocolate sometimes or a large portion of something I really like. But I do not make a habit of it. And I always exercise three times a week.

I have given all my old clothes to the needy. I am committed to never going back to my old ways. That is commitment and that is my secret.

Bart D.

And studies have shown that breakfast eaters are the most fit, have more energy, and burn more calories throughout the day.

The best way to keep yourself from eating more than you need is to feed yourself before you get famished. I'm a big believer in having six mini-meals a day so that you're getting between 200 and 400 calories every three to four hours. See chapter 4 for meal suggestions.

Bad Habit #4: *Getting Into an Exercise Rut*

Your body is smart. If you do the same exercise every day, your muscles will learn how to be more and more efficient in their movements. It gets easier and easier to do what used to be difficult. Efficient movement, however, doesn't burn as many calories as an activity you're not as accustomed to.

So variety is important. Changing your activities will help your body burn more calories and keep your attitude fresh.

Do the same workout day in and day out and your body will be as bored as your mind. Try to incorporate new moves into your routine every six weeks or so. Chapters 7 through 10 offer workouts for strength, flexibility, core stability, and cardio fitness so you can challenge your body in new ways whenever you need to.

DON'T LOSE YOUR PATIENCE

It's incredibly difficult to get rid of all your misconceptions, excuses, and bad habits all at once. So be kind to yourself and work on improving or correcting one thing at a time.

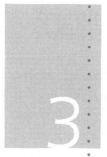

Operation Motivation:
Building a Better Body Image

3

Motivation is what gets you started.
Habit is what keeps you going.
—JIM RYAN, THREE-TIME OLYMPIC ATHLETE

Are you feeling either depressed or deprived? If this question resonates with you, you are not alone. Just about every woman I know struggles with her own personal energy crisis. Women are generous with their energy: They give until there's nothing left. And then they feel bad because they don't have anything more to offer!

"Are you depressed or deprived?" is a question I ask my clients all the time. If you spend your days on the run—running your home, your career, your kids to all their activities—and you don't take the time to replenish yourself with the rest, nourishment, and exercise you need, you're going to run out.

So what happens when you run out, when you don't have the energy and the resources to maintain your schedule? Maybe you turn to sugar and caffeine, hoping that the quick hits of energy will allow you to cruise through whatever immediate crisis you're facing. Unfortunately, the short-term energy surge will always take a greater toll, leaving you even more depleted. It's borrowed energy and your body knows you're going to have to pay it back with interest.

Or perhaps you turn on yourself, angry that you can't do everything you think you should be doing. You call yourself lazy and undisciplined and criticize yourself harshly. With each so-called failure, you punish yourself and resolve to be stricter next time. Initially, on the first few days of an extreme diet or a rigorous exercise program, you feel better, like you're more in control. But it never lasts. Strictness always fails to deliver the perfection it promises. You end up in a perpetual state of adolescent rebellion against your own impossible standards.

In either case, these coping strategies are just distractions and they are never going to give you what you want in the long run. You won't get what you want until you give yourself what you need.

THE SECRETS TO SELF-ACCEPTANCE

What does it mean to nurture yourself? Nurturing is different from indulgence. Indulgence means eating a pint of ice cream. Nurturing means fixing yourself a delicious, balanced meal and taking the time to enjoy not only how good it tastes, but also how good it makes you feel.

Nurture is the kind, generous care you'd give to a child whom you love. It means being gentle when she needs to be corrected and firm when she needs to be protected.

Nurturing means taking care of yourself mentally, physically, and spiritually. It means trying something you've always wanted to do, even if that means taking a risk. Take risks, even if they make you afraid. It's not wrong to feel fear, but you have so much to lose if you let your fears make all your decisions for you. Remember, there is no such thing as a mistake. Mistakes are lessons that we learn from; they make us better, wiser people. I know it can be hard to put aside our insecurities, but sometimes, when we face our fears, we gain the most.

In the fifteen years I've been doing this, I have grown to understand the people who are fully committed versus those who are full of excuses. There is a difference, and it manifests as self-control, self-commitment, and self-respect. Over the years, I have had clients who can't seem to make that commitment. They cancel appointments frequently; they complain about time and, quite frankly, sabotage themselves. They just aren't ready to change.

Then there are clients who are driven, who have a passion to change their lives and are willing to do the planning and make the effort. I help them stay on track, but they do the work. Yes, they can get impatient sometimes, but their overall big-picture perspective tells them to stick with it and persevere.

Genetics do play a part in our health and weight. But that is not an excuse: It's even more of a reason to care. Trying to look like a model or a movie star is an unrealistic goal. What you see in fashion and celebrity magazines—and even some fitness magazines—is unattainable for most of us, and even more unattainable as we age. Models have great lighting and great makeup. Their images are often airbrushed and sometimes digitally altered. Without these tricks of the trade, even models don't always look like models!

Media images are designed to catch our eye and sell us products. Unfortunately, those images make us feel bad; they become intertwined with our self-esteem. We measure ourselves against these unattainable ideals and always come up short. But the body type of a bikini model does not have to be the only goal you have for yourself. How about happiness, health, confidence, energy, and muscle tone? These are attainable—and valuable—at any age.

Those of us who are mothers know that you don't always feel glamorous when you are wiping noses, scrubbing out stains, and washing grubby fingers. It's so important to remember to look for beauty within. Personally, as I age, I've come to believe that the less makeup, the better. Even when I'm wearing sweats, my hair's in a ponytail, and my face is bare, I still feel beautiful. It's what's inside that emanates.

THE AGE OF ENLIGHTENMENT

We don't have to give up on beauty when we bid farewell to youth. Beauty as we age is different: It comes from the inside but it's absolutely visible on the outside. When you are strong and serene, you are beautiful. I know lots of women who feel better at forty than they did at twenty. They have more control of their lives. Their emotions and their appearance improve.

I also know many wise, accomplished, and fabulous women who struggle. They have appetite cravings. They feel tired and worn down.

A Role Model for Mid-Life

After years of struggling with her body—and her mind—Laura Duffek finally realized that the elusive secrets she was seeking were neither elusive nor secret!

"If you're not going to eat right and exercise today, then what? What are you going to do to take control of your life?" That was one of the most powerful questions I have ever been asked in my life. Chris Freytag is the one person who made me stop and think about the consequences of not being committed to a healthy lifestyle. And she has helped me change my life!

I have spent so much time dieting, unhappy, and constantly searching for a magic way to easily lose weight and change my body. At forty, I still hadn't found the "trick" to change everything.

My battle with the bulge has not been a privately fought war. As a television host, I work in front of millions of viewers every day who witnessed my yo-yo dieting. I felt embarrassed and tired of trying everything only to remain overweight. Chris's reply to my whining and pessimistic attitude was: "Get over yourself!" She told me that we were going to work on this together, that the tools were at my disposal, and that I had to want to do it. If I need help, she is there for me. Chris offers a realistic attitude with the strength to motivate and the guiding hand to help me over my challenges.

To say that Chris changed my way of thinking is an understatement. I've listened to her commonsense approach and, forty pounds later, am happier and smarter about living a healthier lifestyle. And every day I still ask myself: "If I don't eat right and exercise today, then how am I going to achieve my goals?"

Their waistlines and hips are expanding, even if they eat less. Their skin, hair, and hormones are changing. They have overloaded brains, overloaded schedules, and never enough hours in the day. If you are concerned about having these feelings, relax, you are absolutely normal. Hopefully, as we all age, we will learn the wisdom of letting go of the "Superwoman" image.

I breezed through my twenties, eating desserts and drinking alcohol and never worrying about my weight or cellulite. However, my body started to change around age thirty. I began to become more concerned with longevity and my body's health. I had three kids and noticed the toll it took on my time, emotions, and appearance. Today I'm actively concerned with my health and try to make good food and exercise choices by treating myself with respect. I am careful about sunscreen, alcohol intake, and sugar. And I work out almost every day—not only because it's my job, but also because I love it. It makes me feel great, and it's important to my health and mental well-being.

I'm not perfect but I do practice what I preach. When I have less time on my hands, I just do what I can. If I'm traveling I'll do push-ups, Pilates, and yoga in my hotel room. Some days I only get to power walk for ten minutes on my treadmill; other days I teach two hours of class. Yes, my life gets crazy. But I still make careful, conscious, and educated decisions when I'm on the go.

I am a realist, so I understand it's important to acknowledge that health issues tend to surface with age. Because I'm starting from a position of strength, I am not afraid to face them and press on. Illness can be difficult and unfortunately not always curable, but that is life and we must appreciate what we have right now! Why not preserve it and live at your potential while you can?

Some people view aging with despair. I view it as a gift. The other day, I was on the phone with a friend and we were discussing how crazy our lives are, how impossible it is to get everything done. She said, "When things feel out of control, I always tell myself, 'It's a great day when it's another day above ground!'"

Which brings up another point: Staying in touch with friends and loved ones, even if they're miles away, is so important to your mental and emotional health. Caring for others and knowing how much they care about you is always good medicine.

OVERCOMING SETBACKS AND DISCOURAGEMENT

Remember the saying "Find the good in the bad." Look at the big picture. Sometimes we get so caught up in the small details that we lose focus of the overall goal or big picture. So much of your success

A Fresh Start at Sixty

My Aunt Mary Kay is proof that you're never too old to change your life. This is her story:

Two years ago, at age fifty-eight, I was totally out of shape and tired. I had no motivation. I spent time with Chris over the holiday season and became absolutely inspired. I decided that, by the time I turned sixty, I would be fit and proud to tell people my age.

I cannot tell you how many times in the last two years it would have been easy to curl up on the couch with my dog and eat bonbons. But then I would remember Chris and tell myself, "Only ten minutes." I would get going and ten minutes would turn into an hour—many times an hour and a half. It became a way of life.

Now, at age sixty, I am twenty-five pounds lighter and I live a life of energy. Everyday activities like housework and gardening are easier. And my brain is functioning better: I don't forget things and it's easier to make decisions.

Thank you, Chris!

Love,

Aunt MK

or failure depends on how you think. The healthy lifestyle game is all about mindfulness, about making changes in your thinking that help keep you going. In actuality, health and fitness is a three-part plan: It's what you do, what you eat, and what you think! And what you think is the most important component of the three—because the other two depend on it.

THE THREE UNBEARABLES: GUILT, FEAR, AND REGRET

Are you constantly reliving past mistakes, wishing you'd had better opportunities, or worrying about things that haven't happened yet? If so, has stewing over these things ever solved anything? I call it the "woulda, coulda, shoulda" problem—and it won't go away on its own.

Guilt, fear, and regret are just thoughts. But if you let them dictate the way you live, you're never going to be happy with the results.

KEEP PERSPECTIVE

While I advocate goal-setting and planning, gorging on extreme details won't make you thin. I've learned not to bog down my clients with every small fact of health and fitness. It's funny because I am such a type A, "give me more information" kind of person. I know a lot about nutrition that is interesting and useful for some applications, like peak athletic performance and bodybuilding competitions. However, is it applicable to my normal client with the goals of better health, more toned muscles, and a more rewarding lifestyle? Probably not!

There is so much information out there and so many rules, you can become completely overwhelmed by the scientific details. Sometimes clients will ask me questions like "Am I allowed to eat fruit and protein in the same meal?" Whoa! Does that really matter when you're trying to lose thirty pounds? Really, the bottom line is that you have to eat less and eat healthy, so if you incorporate these guidelines into your diet, go ahead and eat fruit with some lean protein.

You don't have to obsess over what's happening in every cell of your body. Focus instead on how many calories you eat and how many you expend. It's the simple, reasonable, and sensible kind of common knowledge that will serve you well on your road to better health.

Top Mood Improvers

It's hard maintaining a healthy lifestyle when you're busy with working, parenting, errands, and travels. Does adding "get into shape" to your to-do list seem impossible? You can create and maintain your motivation with inspiration:

- Reread your journal; you'll feel proud about what you've accomplished.

- Try a program of three mini-workouts a day when your life feels out of control. A quick power walk in the evening can relieve stress and help take your mind off the ice cream in the freezer.

- Take the ice cream out of the freezer. If it makes you feel bad to have temptation so close at hand, get rid of it! It's better to "waste it" by throwing it away than to throw it into your body.

- Buy a smoothie maker. Experiment with new combinations, try some exotic fruits, sip through a straw, and relax with a book!

- Laugh! Read a funny story, turn on the comedy channel, or share jokes with your kids or your spouse.

- Join a gym and meet your friends there. Take a group exercise class and sweat it out with others!

- Eat breakfast: You'll be surprised what it does for your mood. See how good it feels to start the day with energy and a focused mind!

- Dance and sing. When people are asked, "What do you do when no one is looking," a large majority say they dance or sing. So turn on the tunes, sing your heart out, and shake your booty!

- Take a bubble bath. When I've had a really bad day, getting into the tub feels so good.

- Treat yourself to a massage. It's one of the best ways to release tension and toxins.

It isn't absolutely necessary to pay a personal trainer or dietician to sort this all out. Of course, if you can afford it, it's great to have someone to cheer you on and steer you in the right direction. But ultimately, it's not about whom you hire but whom you are willing to become—by using common sense, being honest with yourself, and making the commitment to change!

Are you a glass-half-full optimist or a glass-half-empty pessimist? In my experience, negative thinking has never helped anyone to achieve his or her dreams.

PATIENCE COMES WITH PRACTICE

One of the most exasperating things about losing weight the right and safe way is that the loss of two pounds a week isn't always noticed right away by friends and family. If the compliments aren't flying in your direction at first—and please remember this when you get discouraged—you may need to give it eight to twelve weeks before someone notices that you are looking better. They may notice right away your new attitude or your new habits, but your body changes take time. The good news about these slow-to-be-noticed changes is that they are much more likely to be permanent. The weight loss you achieve on a two-week crash diet is an illusion, and the pounds will all come back in the next month. But when you lose the slow and sensible way, those are real pounds and real inches lost, real habits formed, and real lifestyle changes that make you a different person.

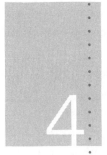

Fuel Efficiency:
Eating to Lose

4

Tell me what you eat and I will tell you what you are.

—BRILLAT-SAVARIN

Weekly I appear on ShopNBC to talk to viewers about a variety of health and fitness topics. But one aspect of my message doesn't vary at all. Just about every week, my viewers will hear me say, at least once:

It's about calories in versus calories out.

This is actually good news for people who are struggling with their weight because it's really very simple. It all comes down to basic arithmetic. If you eat 2,000 calories today and you burn 2,250, you're losing weight. If you eat the same 2,000 calories but you only burn 1,800 because you had a very sedentary day or your metabolism has slowed down from the deprivations of dieting, you're gaining weight. Yes, this is a simplification. There is more to it: hormones, genetics, and medications you may be taking. But these are things we can't control, and worrying about them will just make us crazy. That's why I focus on calories in and calories out. It's the bottom line.

Every extra pound on your body represents 3,500 extra calories that you consumed but did not need. To lose that extra pound, you have to create a 3,500-calorie deficit. And the best way to create a calorie deficit is to eat a little bit less and burn a little bit more by moving your body. It's simple. It's slow. It doesn't have to be boring. But it's the best way to do it.

I tell my clients to budget their calories like they budget their money. We give our children an allowance and encourage them to think about how they want to spend it. Think about your daily calories like a daily allowance: Are you going to get enough pleasure and satisfaction out of a doughnut that it's worth spending 250 calories? Or would you rather save those 250 calories and spend them on something else that would make you happier?

In this chapter, we're going to talk about how to eat a little bit less without depriving yourself of the two things food can give you: nutrients and pleasure. Food is not your enemy. Lack of movement is. So get moving and eat better and you'll achieve a happier, healthier lifestyle.

CALCULATING CALORIES

Although there are very complicated formulas you can use to determine precisely how many calories you need to eat each day to maintain your weight based on your gender and your age, most people simply don't have that kind of time. So I recommend the following shortcut:

Step 1:   Multiply your weight by 10.

Step 2:   Add 20 to 40 percent if you are sedentary.

Add 40 to 60 percent if you are moderately active.

Add 60 to 80 percent if you are very active.

The total is the number of calories you should consume daily.

Example: For a woman who weighs 140 pounds:

140 x 10   = 1,400 calories

1,400 x 1.20   = 1,680 calories

1,400 x 1.40   = 1,960 calories

1,400 x 1.60   = 2,240 calories

1,400 x 1.80   = 2,520 calories

This will give you a good, approximate range for the daily calories your body needs to maintain your current weight. To lose weight slowly and safely, keep your daily calorie intake at the low end of the range for your activity level. If you are extremely overweight, this formula may overestimate your needed calories. Consult your doctor for an appropriate goal weight to use.

You don't have to count calories every day—but when starting a new and healthier lifestyle, it's important to get an accurate sense of how much food you need versus how much you're actually consuming. Calculating your calories is much easier than counting "net" carbs, counting fat grams, or keeping track of complicated rules about food combining. The low-carb craze has put most Americans into a state of "calorie denial." Recent studies have shown that a large percentage of Americans truly believe that they can lose weight by cutting carbs and not cutting calories. In addition, many believe that portion control doesn't matter as long as you cut out the carbs. However, I still go back to the energy equation. To lose weight, it's calories in versus calories out.

CLEAN EATING

I'm not a nutritionist and I don't create specific food plans for my personal training clients. I believe the best food strategy is a well-planned, well-informed menu that you create yourself, because you can customize it to work with the rhythms of your day and include the foods you like to eat.

Instead, I educate my clients in what I call "clean eating." Clean eating is simple. It means that you try to eat things that come from plants, animals, or trees instead of boxes, bags, and take-out containers. It means that you aim to get the majority of your calories from fresh fruits and vegetables, minimally processed grains like whole-wheat bread, low-fat dairy, brown rice, lean meats and fish, nuts, and seeds.

The problem with foods that come in boxes and bags is that they are rich in things your body doesn't need: preservatives to prolong shelf life, sodium to make it taste good, chemically altered fats to make it moist and chewy, and artificial colors to make it look as good as fresh food. These foods are often deficient in things your body needs, like fiber, which keeps you regular and helps you feel full and satisfied.

Clean eating also means that you try to get a variety of foods into each meal—some protein, some grains, some fruit or vegetables—and that you aim to eat a variety of meals each week. Many people find themselves

A Clean Eating Testimonial

Clean eating can make a dramatic difference in the health of your body, and Jill S. is living proof. Here's how she lowered her cholesterol and changed her life!

Last August I happened to mention to Chris that I had just had my cholesterol checked, and for the fourth year in a row, it was over 200! I told her that despite my efforts to lower it, nothing seemed to help. I had cut out beef and animal fat and I was not eating much butter or dairy. But it was when I told her my family history that she said, "That's it, you're only thirty-eight and we want you around for a long time." Three out of four of my grandparents died of heart attacks. My dad has had a heart attack and a stroke and today has a pacemaker. My mom has had two strokes and is on medication for both high blood pressure and cholesterol.

Chris said we had to evaluate everything I ate and see what was out of whack. She invited me over to her house and we discussed my diet. I tended to eat fat-free snacks to cut back on cholesterol—things like packaged Rice Krispie treats, baked chips, chewy granola bars, etc. For several hours, Chris educated me on "trans fats." Who would have thought—with a cholesterol problem like mine—that no one ever told me about the danger of partially hydrogenated oils. She laid out her whole program of clean eating: being conscious of whether foods come from a plant or animal. She really taught me about what I should and shouldn't be eating. The long and short of it: no hydrogenated oils. I thought I was being good by having baked chips and crackers, but they're all full of trans fats. I even changed my wheat bread.

I basically wiped my kitchen clean and went to the grocery store the next day. I just started reading labels and found foods I love without it. I educated my three kids, and we started eating differently. It wasn't very hard and really my kids didn't even complain. We found lots of options and I started cutting up apples instead of always eating prepackaged stuff!

It is now six months later and I just had my cholesterol levels rechecked. I told Chris I was nervous to see if my cholesterol had gone down, because if it hadn't, it may be time for medication! Sure enough, my cholesterol went from 237 to 185, and my triglycerides went from 188 to 66. Not only that, but, I went from a size 12 to a size 8 without even dieting! I just started eating less packaged foods and eating more fresh foods. Chris knows her stuff, and I'm so grateful that she sat me down that day because I learned so much and maybe lengthened my life!

eating the same things for lunch and dinner over and over again because it's easy.

In essence, clean eating means eating food that's free of heavy sauces and sweeteners. It means eating fruit rather than juice, as the fruit contains fiber and some nutrients not present in the juice. It means eating five servings of fruits and vegetables a day.

Clean eating does not mean perfect eating. It doesn't mean that you'll never ever see a cookie or a bag of potato chips again. As anyone who has ever spent five minutes on a diet can tell you, the best way to create a craving out of thin air is to declare that a food like chocolate or bread is forbidden. (This doesn't work on broccoli or tofu—I don't know why. It just doesn't.)

Practicing clean eating at home means buying fresh produce at the supermarket—and then actually using it. It means gently and gradually introducing healthy substitutions to your family's meals, such as ground turkey meatballs instead of ground beef, or brown rice instead of white rice. It doesn't mean cooking elaborate meals that take hours to prepare. In chapter 5, you'll find simple meal ideas that let you feed your family and have a life at the same time.

Clean eating at restaurants means asking for sauces to be served on the side. It means asking to have meats broiled or grilled instead of fried. It means asking for extra vegetables as a substitute for creamy, buttery mashed potatoes with gravy. It means knowing that you have the right, as a restaurant customer, to ask for what you want.

Clean eating at holiday gatherings is about making small, satisfying exceptions to the rules. It's better to eat a small scoop of stuffing or a little sliver of pie than to feel deprived and left out.

PORTION CONTROL

A recent study at the University of North Carolina confirmed that serving sizes in the United States are expanding as fast as the American waistline. Researchers analyzed portion sizes over a twenty-year period. Here's a sampling of the smorgasbord they found:

- Hamburgers grew 23 percent between 1977 and 1996.
- Soft-drink serving sizes increased by 52 percent.
- Servings of snack foods, such as chips and pretzels, were 60 percent larger.

The reason behind these giant meals is marketing. Food marketers discovered that consumers perceived larger quantities as better values for their money. So offering big servings has become a proven marketing technique: You buy more because you believe you're getting a better deal.

If you really wanted to get precise about portions, you could carry around a set of measuring cups and a kitchen scale so you can weigh and measure every bite. But you're already equipped with a convenient food measurement device. You're using it right now to hold this book. You can use your hand to estimate portion sizes pretty accurately.

- The size of your fist   =   A medium fruit, one cup of rice or pasta
- The size of your thumb   =   One ounce of cheese
- The tip of your thumb   =   One teaspoon of butter, oil, or nut butter
- The palm of your hand   =   One serving of meat, poultry, or fish
- One cupped handful   =   One serving of cereal, chips, or pretzels

Try it the next time you go out for lunch. You'll be surprised to see just how much food you have on your hands!

THE NUTRIENTS YOU NEED

Your body needs three kinds of nutrients to function well: protein, carbohydrates, and fats. We'll focus on these primary nutrients, rather than getting into specifics about vitamins and minerals, because the "big three" are the nutrients that concern most dieters—and diet designers.

Some diet fads blame weight gain on fat consumption or carbohydrate consumption. This is misleading. If you take in too many calories—regardless of whether they're fat calories, carbohydrate calories, or protein calories—the result is always the same: You'll gain weight.

To figure out how much protein, carbohydrate, and fat are contained in the foods you eat, check the Nutrition Facts box on the package or label. For foods that don't come with labels, you can find several pocket-sized nutrition reference books at most bookstores.

Protein

Protein is your body's building material. Your body needs protein to build and repair muscle, bone, and cartilage. Your body can't store protein for the long term so you need to consume protein in your diet every day. Foods rich in protein include meats, poultry, fish, dairy products, eggs, nuts, and legumes such as soybeans and kidney beans. Protein contains four calories per gram. I advise my clients to consume between 0.5 and 0.8 grams of protein per pound of body weight per day. Aim for 0.8 grams per pound per day if you are consistently strength training; otherwise 0.5 grams per pound is plenty. For example, a 130-pound woman should try to eat approximately 65 grams of protein per day, give or take.

Carbohydrate

Carbohydrates are your body's immediate energy supply. They come in two varieties: simple carbohydrates, which are sugars, and complex carbohydrates. Complex carbohydrates are slowly broken down into sugars in your small intestine so that they can be used to fuel your muscles, nerves, and brain. Generally speaking, complex carbohydrates from grains and vegetables are better for your body than sugars and refined carbs, which are broken down too quickly into sugar.

Sugars—found in soft drinks, candies, and sweetened baked goods like cake and cookies—rush to the bloodstream, providing fast energy that disappears quickly. Complex carbohydrates enter the bloodstream more slowly, creating less dramatic surges in your blood sugar.

The typical American pantry is filled with refined carbohydrate foods, such as white-flour breads and crackers, which are high on the glycemic index. This means that they cause a rapid rise in blood sugar. Your body responds by releasing a lot of insulin, a hormone secreted by the pancreas. The insulin causes your blood sugar to plummet, which makes you hungry again. These dramatic ups and downs affect your energy, your mood, and your waistline.

Like protein, carbohydrates contain four calories per gram. To maintain balanced nutrition during weight loss, about 40 percent of your total daily calories should come from quality complex carbohydrates. If you consume 2,000 calories per day (a figure that is considered sufficient for an average, healthy, active woman who is not trying to lose weight), you need about 200 grams of carbohydrates. For those who are moving to lose, and are consuming, say, 1,500 calories per day, that would equal a carb intake of about 150 grams.

Foods rich in complex carbohydrates are also more likely to be rich in fiber. Fiber isn't a nutrient but it is a necessary part of your diet. Fiber is the indigestible plant material contained in edible grains and vegetables. Fiber makes food more satisfying because it takes up space, helping you to feel full faster. And it slows digestion, which delays the onset of hunger pangs. Because fiber doesn't break down in the digestive process, it also helps to sweep waste through your body. Fiber-rich foods include whole grains (to determine if a food is whole grain, ensure that *whole* wheat or some other *whole* grain is listed as the first ingredient on the ingredients list; don't be fooled by misleading label terminology—"unbleached wheat flour" is not whole wheat), vegetables, fruits, and legumes. Twenty-five grams of fiber per day is the standard for healthy digestion and absorbs up to 200 calories. If you're adding fiber to your diet, do so gradually to give your body time to adjust.

Fat

Fat is your body's long-term energy supply. It contains nine calories per gram, making it more than twice as calorie rich as protein or carbohydrates. Fat also makes you feel full and satisfied. Your body needs fat to provide energy reserves, maintain body heat, and protect you from injuring bones and muscles.

There are several kinds of fats. Saturated fats are animal fats like butter and beef fat that stay solid at room temperature. Diets rich in saturated fat increase your risk of plaque buildup in your coronary arteries, which leads to heart disease. Doctors tell their patients that the harder the fat, the more it blocks the arteries.

Monounsaturated and polyunsaturated fats, such as most vegetable oils, are liquid at room temperature. These, in moderation, are the good-for-you fats, such as olive and canola oils. Other good sources of healthy fats are peanuts, almonds, nut butters, avocados, and seeds such as pumpkin and sunflower.

Unsaturated fats can be artificially processed to remain solid at room temperature. This process is called hydrogenation. You'll find hydrogenated fats, also known as trans fats, in margarines and shortenings. Makers of processed foods began using these fats in their products several decades ago to lengthen their shelf life. These man-made fats also help crackers stay crisp and add an appealing chewy texture to cookies and granola bars. Recent research, however, has revealed that these fats are even unhealthier than saturated fats. Diets high in hydrogenated and partially hydrogenated fats raise your bad (LDL) cholesterol level and deplete the good cholesterol (HDL) in your bloodstream, which protects you from heart disease. If an ingredient listing includes any vegetable oils that are hydrogenated or "partially hydrogenated," you're better off without it.

Because fats are calorie dense, containing nine calories per gram, dieters frequently avoid them. But your body needs to get at least a little fat every day. A no-fat diet will leave you with dry skin, lifeless hair, and an insatiable craving for deep-fried anything. Some fats, in moderation, are actually very good for you.

For cooking and baking, my first choice is canola oil. It contains omega-3 fatty acids, which help reduce blood pressure, "bad" LDL cholesterol, and triglyceride levels. My typical salad dressing is either olive or canola oil, vinegar (usually white wine), Dijon mustard, and a little minced garlic and dill. I'll drizzle that over a salad of apples (or grapes), mixed greens, and slivered almonds. And I use it instead of butter or margarine to bake muffins or pop popcorn.

For other salads and savory dishes, I use olive oil. Olive oil contains omega-6 fatty acids and more than thirty different antioxidants, which can help protect heart health and may reduce the risk of cancer. Try drizzling some good-quality extra-virgin olive oil on bread as a substitute for butter. You can sauté vegetables in a little olive oil with a clove of chopped garlic. Or I like to make a healthy version of French fries by cutting fresh potatoes into narrow strips, brushing them lightly with olive oil, sprinkling them with a little kosher salt, and roasting them in a 400-degree oven until they're tender or crisp, depending on what you like.

Many of my fat-phobic clients are surprised when I recommend nuts as a healthy snack. Almonds, peanuts, pecans, and walnuts contain monounsaturated fats that,

Try This Challenge

Go into your kitchen and pick out five snack foods. Search the ingredients labels for partially hydrogenated fats or oils. You'll probably be shocked by how many you find, even in bread! Fortunately, help is on the way. By 2006, the FDA will require that all fact tables on nutrition labels indicate the presence of trans fats.

My Top Favorite Snacks

10

1. Make your own tortilla chips! Use organic flour or corn tortillas, cut into wedges, and bake at 350 degrees for approximately ten minutes or until crisp. Serve with salsa.

2. Celery dipped in peanut butter.

3. High-fiber cereal mixed with toasted sliced almonds; I measure out one cup into a baggie and take it with me when I'm on the go.

4. A bowl of blueberries with one cup of soymilk.

5. Piña colada protein shake: Mix protein powder, pineapple, skim milk, coconut extract, and ice; blend until creamy.

6. Chocolate coffee frozen drink: Mix chocolate-flavored protein powder, vanilla yogurt, ice, and coffee; blend until creamy (just like the coffeehouse favorite but loaded with protein instead of sugar).

7. Tuna salad: Mix tuna fish, low-fat cottage cheese, Dijon mustard, and dill weed; serve on apple slices or wrap in romaine lettuce leaves.

8. Oat and honey granola bar dipped in light strawberry yogurt.

9. Sliced red peppers dipped in hummus.

10. Hot-air popcorn, misted with olive oil, sprinkled with seasoning salt.

when substituted for other fatty foods, can lower "bad" LDL cholesterol, reduce the risk of heart disease, and perhaps also lower the risk of diabetes. Try using finely chopped nuts as a substitute for breading on a sautéed fish filet.

Flaxseed is another one of my favorite sources for healthy fats. Flaxseed is rich in alpha-linolenic acid, the omega-3 fatty acid that helps control inflammation and blood pressure. I sprinkle flaxseed into salads, soups, and spaghetti sauce. And I substitute ground flaxseed for half the oil in baking recipes.

LIQUID CALORIES

Just because they go down easy doesn't mean they don't count. Caloric beverages aren't as filling as food, so they're easy to overdo. A large, sweetened mocha from your favorite coffeehouse made with whipped cream can cost you between 500 and 800 calories. Sports drinks can also be a pitfall. People drink these because they seem healthy. However, unless you're an athlete who engages regularly in strenuous activity, these are simply a source of unnecessary calories. Some can have as many sugary calories as soda. Substitute water or lightly sweetened tea instead.

Alcoholic beverages can be another source of hidden calories. And, since most of them contain no nutritional value, the typical cocktail party is a minefield of empty calories. Like other indulgences, alcohol is usually fine in moderation. If you're on your way to a party, set a goal before you arrive—for example, limit yourself to two glasses of wine, with glasses of water in between. Don't beat yourself up if you overindulge on rare occasions. Just recommit yourself to your healthy lifestyle and keep on going.

MINI-MEALS FOR MAXI-SATISFACTION

I strongly advocate a meal plan of five to six mini-meals a day. It's what I recommend to my clients, and it's how I eat.

Mini-meals help you succeed on both mental and physical levels. Psychologically, mini-meals help you resist unexpected temptations—not to mention the obligatory Monday-morning pastries at the office—by reassuring you that your next healthy, tasty, satis-fying opportunity to eat is just around the corner.

On a physical level, eating small amounts every two to three hours helps to keep your blood sugar on an even keel, making you less susceptible to cravings and food cues like television ads. There's even some scientific ev-idence that indicates that frequent, small meals help you to burn calories at a higher rate because the absence of prolonged hunger prevents your body from turning down your metabolic thermostat to conserve energy.

COMMON SENSE VERSUS THE HOTTEST DIET TRENDS

There are a lot of diet gurus out there and all the competing claims and theories are causing a lot of confusion. But clean eating is sound and sen-sible nutritional advice. Here's how clean eating compares to all the trendy diet fads.

Food Fad	Clean Eating
Grazing: Eating frequently throughout the day to prevent fluctuations in blood sugar and intense cravings. Not a bad idea but tends to easily devolve into continuous snacking without any plan-ning, which can lead to eating too many calories.	**Mini-meals:** Planning your portions gives you a way to measure your success!
Food combining: The theory that some foods should not be eaten at the same time as other foods can be so complicated you have to carry a rulebook at all times!	**Balanced meals:** You need to eat a combination of proteins, good fats, and good carbohydrates at each meal to get a good nutritional foundation. A bal-anced meal, consisting of sensible por-tions, is more satisfying, more nutritious, and more interesting.
Low fat: Dieters who over-restrict fat invariably replace it with sugar, salts, and refined flour products to make up for the lack of satisfaction in their food.	**Good fat:** We understand that fat is really not as disastrous to our diet as it was once believed. Healthy fats can help you feel full and satisfied, and aid in weight loss.

Food Fad	Clean Eating
Carb cutting: Eliminating a total food group from your diet is never a good idea. Carbohydrates are actually a needed source of energy for your body. The real problem with carbohydrates is that we eat too many of the wrong ones, especially sugar.	**Good carbs:** Whole grains and fibrous fruits and vegetables are necessary and nutritious parts of any food plan.
Fast weight loss: Crash diets trick your body into starvation mode and your metabolism slows down.	**Slow weight loss:** You'll lose more fat and maintain muscle if you take a more moderate approach and change your habits slowly. Develop a realistic eating plan, and make food choices that you can stick with for life.

THE FOOD STRATEGY

You can't drive your car to work if it doesn't have any gas in it. The same thing goes for your body. You're not going to get very far if you don't give it any fuel. Dieters often try to skimp on calories by skipping breakfast. Resist the temptation, even if you're not hungry in the morning. Breakfast gives your body the fuel it needs to burn the fat you're trying to lose.

Have your breakfast as soon as possible in the morning. Then try to eat every three to four hours throughout the day so that you have just enough time between meals to feel a little hungry.

I strongly advise against skipping meals to "save" calories that you can spend later on a big pizza or a holiday dinner. I try to encourage my clients to treat themselves at least as well as they treat their cars. You can't put a month's worth of gas into your car just because you don't like to go to the gas station. So don't try to consume a day's worth of calories in one sitting. I warn my clients against what I call the overstuffing principle. Your body simply cannot properly and efficiently use too many calories at once. Anything your body can't use is stored as fat. So binge eaters who starve all day, then gorge, are doing themselves no favors.

I wish we would care for ourselves as well as we care for our pets. I wouldn't dream of serving my dog two days' worth of food in a single feeding. We feed our pets on a schedule that works for their bodies—and we should do the same for ourselves.

The following serving guidelines and eating schedules will help you create small meals that are satisfying without stuffing yourself.

THE CLEAN EATING FOOD PLAN

This plan will come to approximately 1,400 to 1,800 calories per day, which is a safe, doable weight-loss plan for women. Depending on how active you are, you may need more calories. Men can add one or two additional servings of protein, one or two additional servings of grains, and one additional serving of fats.

Basically, this is good, balanced nutrition with real foods and a heaping helping of common sense. You'll be limiting your fats and the less desirable carbohydrate foods, and eating plenty of fruits and veggies, whole grains, and low-fat proteins.

The food lists below identify Best-Better-Bad choices for each food group. For best results, eat primarily from the "Best" choices. You can opt for a "Better" choice once in a while.

Per Day Allowances

Six to eight servings of proteins: One serving = one ounce of meat, seafood, or soy; one cup skim milk or soymilk; one scoop protein powder; two egg whites or ¼ cup egg substitute; one ounce of cheese

Four to six servings of vegetables: One serving = one cup of most cooked veggies, ½ cup of starchy veggies, ¼ cup of tomato sauce or salsa, one cup of raw veggies, unlimited lettuce (dark green lettuces are far more nutritious than iceberg lettuce), unlimited leafy greens, or ½ cup vegetable juice

Two to three servings of fruit: One serving = one medium apple, pear, or banana; one cup berries, grapes, or sliced fruit; ½ cup juice

Five to six servings of grains, breads, and starches: One serving = one slice whole-grain bread; ½–¾ cup high-fiber, low-sugar cereal (at least three grams of fiber and no more than twelve grams of sugar per serving); ½ cup brown or wild rice, potatoes, sweet potatoes, couscous, or pasta; three cups popcorn, one handful of pretzels

One to two servings of fats and condiments: One serving = one teaspoon of oil, a small handful of nuts, two tablespoons of ketchup; you can use mustard and spices in abundance; ¼ medium avocado, two tablespoons of ground flaxseed, one tablespoon of light mayo or margarine

Eight (or more) glasses of water: One glass = eight ounces of plain water, sparkling water, or herbal tea. Drink an extra glass or two if you are exercising or if the weather is hot. Other liquids—such as juices, sodas, coffees, and tea—don't count.

Clean Eating Food Lists
Proteins

BEST (Choose often)	BETTER (Choose occasionally)	BAD (Choose seldom)
Fish; my favorites are: • Salmon • Halibut • Tuna	Lean beef: • Tenderloin • Flank steak • Roast beef	High-fat cuts of beef
Shellfish	Low-fat cheeses	Breaded or fried meats
Skinless turkey breast	Dark meat chicken or turkey	Whole eggs
Ground turkey and turkey burgers	Pork tenderloin and chops	Full-fat dairy and cheeses
Turkey bacon and sausages	Ham	Bacon and sausage
Skinless chicken breast	Flavored yogurts (many are high in sugar)	Sugary yogurts (often marketed to kids)
Soybeans and tofu	Peanut butter	
Legumes—beans and lentils		
Egg whites or egg substitute		
Low-fat dairy products		
Protein powders		

Veggies

BEST (Choose often)	BETTER (Choose occasionally)	BAD (Choose seldom)
Fresh or frozen: Broccoli Spinach Cauliflower Colored peppers Mushrooms Green beans Carrots Celery Zucchini Tomatoes Leafy greens Artichokes Bamboo shoots Brussels sprouts Cabbage Cucumbers Eggplant Onions Peas Water chestnuts Jicama Pumpkin	Corn* Sweet potatoes* Baked potatoes* Beets* Pickles (high in sodium) Lima beans* Canned vegetables with added oils or sodium Winter squash*	Mashed potatoes or any potato made with lots of butter or cream Any vegetable served with hollandaise or cream sauce Fried potatoes, such as French fries, hash browns, and Tater Tots Any vegetable swimming in butter

* **Starchy vegetables** like potatoes (white and sweet), corn, peas, and lima beans contain about the same amount of carbs and calories as many grain products, therefore some nutritionists think of these foods as bread substitutes instead of as vegetables.

* **Beets** are actually quite good for you, but they have the highest sugar content of any vegetable, even higher than carrots.

Fruits

BEST (Choose often)	BETTER (Choose occasionally)	BAD (Choose seldom)
Apples Apricots Blueberries	Banana Avocado Dates	Candied fruits Fruit canned in syrup, or with other added sugars

BEST (Choose often)	BETTER (Choose occasionally)	BAD (Choose seldom)
Cantaloupe	Prunes	Sugary jams and jellies
Honeydew melon	Raisins	Canned pie filling
Cherries	Fruit juices	"Fruit snacks," which are really candy marketed to kids
Cranberries	Coconut	
Grapefruit	Fruit canned in its own juice	
Grapes	*These are high-calorie fruits.*	
Kiwi fruit		
Mangoes		
Nectarines		
Oranges		
Papaya		
Peaches		
Pears		
Pineapple		
Plums		
Pomegranate		
Raspberries		
Strawberries		
Tangerines		
Watermelon		

Breads, Grains, Starches, and Sugars

BEST (Choose often)	BETTER (Choose occasionally)	BAD (Choose seldom)
Whole-wheat, multigrain breads	Popcorn made on the stove with canola or olive oil	White bread and bagels
Whole-grain cereals	Pretzels or crackers made without partially hydrogenated oils	Bakery items like muffins, scones, donuts
Oats or oatmeal (not sugar-sweetened instant oatmeal packets)		Sugary cereals
Brown rice or wild rice		White pasta
Whole-grain pastas		White rice
Hot air–popped popcorn		Microwaveable popcorn (full of trans fats!)
		White flour
		Cakes, pies, cookies

BEST (Choose often)	BETTER (Choose occasionally)	BAD (Choose seldom)
		Candy
		Fat-free snack foods such as prepackaged cookies, bars, etc.
		Added table sugar in your coffee or on your cereal
		Snack chips, regular and fat-free
		Soda pop (diet soda in moderation is okay)
		Sugary flavor shots in your coffee drinks

Fats (Use sparingly)

BEST (Choose often)	BETTER (Choose occasionally)	BAD (Choose seldom)
Avocados—a fruit with a good deal of fat	Light mayonnaise	Butter
Nuts and seeds	Light cream cheese	Full-fat cream cheese
Olives	Palm fruit oil*	Margarine
Flaxseed—you can buy it preground	Light salad dressing	Bacon and sausage fats
Reduced-fat, trans-free margarines		Sour cream
Canola, olive, peanut, sunflower, safflower, sesame, and walnut oils		Bottled salad dressings
		Half-and-half
		Whipped cream
		Palm kernel oil*
		Full-fat mayonnaise
		Coconut oil

* Palm kernel oil is 83 percent saturated fat. Palm fruit oil (sometimes called "palm oil") contains a healthier balance of polyunsaturated, monounsaturated, and saturated fats. Palm fruit oil also contains natural antioxidants and essential fatty acids.

Treats (Substitute one for a grain/starch serving.)

These are special indulgences for happy occasions and times when you might be feeling deprived.

- A six-ounce glass of wine

- A twelve-ounce light beer

- ½ cup frozen yogurt or ice cream

- Dessert: If you must, split it with someone and only eat half!

- Three ginger snaps, or one graham cracker sheet

- Three Hershey's kisses or a small handful of chocolate chips for a chocolate fix

- One light frozen fudge bar

- A slice of my key lime pie (see below)

FAILING TO PLAN IS PLANNING TO FAIL

The world we live in makes it so easy to make poor food choices. Convenience stores stock their most accessible shelves with an array of easy-to-grab candies and chips. Supermarket aisles offer heat-and-eat meals that can be ready in five or ten minutes. Fast-food merchants offer drive-up windows so you don't even have to get the kids out of the car.

Food marketers know you're starved for time. In fact, they're literally banking on how busy you are. Fight back. It's your money and your life.

Better eating requires better planning. It means knowing yourself well enough to anticipate that you always get hungry while you're running afternoon errands in the car, then planning to bring an apple and a handful of nuts along for the ride.

Better planning starts with a grocery list. Once you're in the store, you're

Chris' Key Lime Pie

This is my kids' favorite dessert, hands down. I make this for parties and company all the time. And it's so delicious, no one would ever guess it's a healthy indulgence.

The crust consists of ten graham crackers (the kind with no hydrogenated oils), three tablespoons of canola oil, and three tablespoons of light maple syrup. Break crackers into crumbs. Use a fork or a pastry cutter to mix in oil and syrup. Press into an eight-inch pie tin. Use wax paper to press the crust into the pan if it's sticking to your fingers. Chill the crust while you make the filling.

The filling consists of ⅓ cup key lime juice, a fifteen-ounce can of fat-free sweetened condensed milk, an eight-ounce tub of light, nondairy whipped topping, and a dash of green food coloring. Stir together with a spoon and spread into the crust. Chill for five to eight hours. Top with fresh strawberries if desired.

at the mercy of all the colorful displays and pretty packages that are designed to persuade you to buy. A list will help you stick with your plan.

It's important to remember that change is challenging. The surest way to get discouraged is to try and overhaul all your eating at once. The smartest way to proceed is to go slowly and change one thing a week. If, for example, you're not in the habit of eating salads, try getting a week's worth of salad fixings. If you're always heading for vending-machine candy bars in the afternoon, try stocking your desk drawer with a week's worth of dried fruit, whole-grain crackers, and nuts so you can have a healthy mini-meal instead.

STARTING AT THE STORE

Your new eating habits don't begin at the table or in your kitchen. Your new healthy diet begins at the grocery store! Here are a few tips to help you navigate the supermarket for clean eating:

- Shop the perimeter of the store first. That's where grocers stock all the good-for-you stuff like produce, dairy, and meats. All the aisles in the center of the store contain the packaged foods: crackers, cookies, chips, and frozen meals.

- In the produce department, buy color. Brighter colors mean better nutrients.

- Buy what's in season and try new things.

- Shop often and buy smaller amounts of perishable produce; most fruit and veggies stay good for about four to five days.

Fishing for Cooking Tips?

So many home cooks suffer from a fear of fish. But the good-for-you benefits of seafood are well worth making an attempt to cook outside of your comfort zone. So-called fatty fish, such as herring, mackerel, salmon, and tuna, deliver plenty of high-quality protein, along with omega-3 fatty acids, which help reduce your risk of heart attack and stroke by lowering blood pressure and cholesterol.

Stress-free Salmon

Brush a filet of salmon with a teaspoon of olive oil. Add a few sprigs of rosemary, dill, or thyme, salt, and pepper, then slow roast or grill until the flesh is opaque.

Simple Shrimp

Boil them quickly or skewer them, brush with olive oil, sprinkle with seasoning salt, and grill until pink. Serve cold or hot, with a lemon wedge or cocktail sauce.

Mediterranean Trout

Brush a filet of trout with olive oil and lemon juice, then coat with seasoned whole-wheat breadcrumbs and bake at 350 degrees until the flesh flakes easily with a fork.

- Set up for the week on Sundays! Pick up basics like chicken breasts and brown rice in quantities that will be enough for two or three meals. You can cook these in advance on Sunday afternoon so you'll be able to make quick dinners on busy weeknights.

- Check ingredient listings: Avoid anything with partially hydrogenated oils, which are often found in breads, cereals, cookies, etc.

- Watch for marbling in meats. A marbled appearance means higher fat.

- At the deli counter, watch out for sodium-laden luncheon meats. Whenever possible, purchase minimally processed, real meats, rather than the processed or pressed versions full of fats, nitrates, and preservatives. Nutritional information is usually available if you ask!

- Buy frozen fruits and veggies. These last a long time and are great when you are in a time crunch. Frozen fruit works well in smoothies. Also stock your freezer with extra chicken breasts, ground turkey, and a spare loaf of whole-grain bread.

- Skip the soda: Try sugar-free flavored waters!

- Watch out for canned or packaged soups and sauces; most are loaded with sodium.

- Stock up on salt-free seasonings. They are delicious and add tons of flavors—you won't even miss the butter.

- I recommend adding butter-flavored sprinkles to your spice rack for those times when you're craving the real thing.

Once you get your groceries home, be sure to store them wisely for maximum freshness and flavor. Refrigeration can help fresh produce last longer but make sure fruits are ripe before you chill them. Keep produce out of the sun! The exception is tomatoes, which are best ripened on a sunny windowsill and should never be refrigerated.

I wash my produce before I put it away so that it's ready when I need it. I just throw it all into one big colander, rinse it thoroughly, and let it dry on clean dishtowels.

CLEANING UP THE KITCHEN

If you followed my advice about grocery shopping, your kitchen should be brimming with easily accessible healthy foods. So right now, while you're awash with resolve to change your life for the better, go through your cupboards and get rid of the bad stuff. If the packages aren't open, donate them to a local food shelter. If it's open, simply pitch it.

No, you are *not* wasting food. Eating stuff that's bad for you is what's truly wasteful.

If you don't have kids, don't sabotage yourself by keeping a few temptations in the house. You can't eat it if you don't have it. If you do have kids, you'll probably have a mutiny on your hands if you clear all the goodies out of your pantry. So just do the best you can to remove the things that trigger your binges.

Feeling a little deprived? Spruce up your spice rack! Treat yourself to fresh batches of your favorites and try a few new flavors to inspire your creativity.

Clean Kitchen Essentials

Treat yourself to some new kitchen gear to make it faster and easier to cook the clean eating way:

- I swear by my mini chopper. This kitchen gadget is great for chopping onions, garlic, fresh herbs, fresh ginger, nuts, and all those labor-intensive ingredients that add real zing to your cooking.

- An olive oil mister is a spray bottle designed to let you refill and pressurize olive oil for quick sprays on cookware or air-popped popcorn.

- A pastry brush helps you add just the lightest layer of oil onto vegetables or fish.

- A blender is an essential for protein smoothies, fruit smoothies, and the fluffiest scrambled eggs.

- Think about investing in a couple of nonstick saucepans and sauté pans so you can brown foods with less fat.

SUPERFOODS: A FEW OF MY FAVORITE THINGS

A Cup of Green Tea

In all my research, I have yet to discover even one negative thing written about green tea. Green tea is reported to be a preventative for all sorts of ailments, including many cancers and heart diseases, and protects your skin, organs, and tissues from the toils of time. It is high in antioxidant polyphenols, which help protect you from heart attack, stroke, and some cancers. Green tea contains about half the caffeine of coffee. I won't give up my cup of coffee in the morning but I'll sip green tea throughout the day. It makes me feel relaxed and energized at the same time!

Cinnamon, the Spice That's Twice as Nice

It's more than a fragrant addition to lattes and cookie recipes: Cinnamon is a natural diuretic, which can help you alleviate excess water weight. Some research suggests that cinnamon may help improve both glucose and cholesterol levels in the blood, which may prove to be useful for diabetics. I sprinkle it on whole-wheat toast or hot oatmeal, mix it into my protein shakes and pancake mix, add a light dusting of it to hot beverages, toss a little of it into hot popcorn, and add it to seasoning rubs for poultry. Cinnamon also is a great addition to bread and muffin recipes.

Rooting for Ginger

Studies show that ginger has some anticancer benefits and can soothe your troubled tummy. It can be helpful in relieving the nausea of pregnancy and motion sickness. A dash of freshly grated ginger root adds a delicious zest to an Asian stir-fry.

Spicy Cayenne

It's not only a popular kitchen spice but a "hot" supplement as well! Adding a sprinkle of cayenne to your meal is an excellent way to stimulate the circulatory system, increasing the supply of blood throughout the body and encouraging the removal of toxins. It can be a digestive aid and some cultures believe it prevents and or diminishes the symptoms of the common cold.

Sweet Stevia

This natural herbal sweetener, which is extracted from the leaves of a plant native to Paraguay, is about three hundred times sweeter than sugar. Although the FDA has not approved stevia for specific use as a sweetener, it is sold as a dietary supplement in natural food stores. You can buy boxes of individual packets for convenience.

Blueberries

Blueberries are a true superfood. They are packed with antioxidants, which can protect you from the free-radical damage that's behind everything from wrinkles to clogged arteries to cancer! When fresh blueberries are out of season, keep your freezer stocked. Frozen blueberries can go straight into smoothies and muffin recipes—no thawing required.

Cranberries

Cranberries are another one of my favorite superfoods. They are widely used to prevent and treat urinary tract infections. We often think of cranberries at Thanksgiving, but cranberries are also powerful antioxidants that protect against heart disease, cancer, and other diseases year-round. Try the tart-sweet taste of dried cranberries in your salad.

The Subtle Sweetness of Brown Rice Syrup

This traditional Asian sweetener is made from fermented brown rice and has a subtle caramel flavor. It resembles honey but is less intense. Try it in marinades and salad dressings or use it as a beverage sweetener. It can be used in baking for items that don't rise, such as cookies.

EASY TO FIX, EASY TO LOVE

Here are a few of my favorite fast recipes that my family loves too!

My Favorite Sloppy Joe Recipe

Brown one pound of lean ground beef or ground turkey. Add ½ cup of chopped onions, ½ cup of ketchup, two tablespoons each of white wine vinegar and Splenda sugar substitute. Add one tablespoon each of yellow mustard and Worcestershire sauce. Simmer and serve on whole-grain buns.

This takes less than ten minutes to make and it's one of my kid's favorites. Serve with some fruit and it's dinner!

My Favorite Pizza Recipe

I start with an organic frozen pizza crust. First, I roll it out and prebake it according to the package directions. Then I spread a thin layer of Thai peanut sauce on the crust and top it with chopped scallions, cubes of cooked chicken breast, and shredded carrots. Bake it at 400 degrees for approximately 10 to 15 minutes.

My Favorite Protein Shake

I mix vanilla protein powder, canned pumpkin, cinnamon, stevia, vanilla soymilk, and ice cubes in my blender for a smoothie that tastes like pumpkin pie without the guilt (or the holiday hassles).

DEAR DIARY

In my experience, there is one thing that separates the people who succeed at clean eating from the people who give up and go back to their old ways. The people who succeed are the people who write down everything they eat when beginning a lifestyle change.

Many people don't want to do a food diary because it takes too much time. But that's actually one of the benefits of using a diary: You're less likely to sneak an extra snack if you don't want to take the time to write it down!

A food diary is the surest cure for mindless eating, which is the most fattening kind of eating there is. Mindless eating is being surprised to discover that you've polished off an entire bag of pretzels while you were watching television. It's "tasting" and nibbling while you're cooking dinner. It's eating the food that your kids didn't finish because you don't want to waste it. Just because you're not paying attention doesn't mean the calories don't count.

Keeping a food diary ensures that every bite you take is a bite you consciously choose to take. You can copy the food diary format on page 61 into a notebook or use it to create a document on your computer that you can customize to suit your own eating habits. If you consume a lot of bites and nibbles one particular day, add a few more spaces.

Food Diary   Date

	Calories	Fat Grams	Carb Grams	Protein Grams
Breakfast				
Snack #1				
Lunch				
Snack #2				
Dinner				
Snack #3				
Totals				

Water (8 to 12 glasses per day) ☐ ☐ ☐ ☐ ☐ ☐ ☐ ☐ ☐ ☐ ☐ ☐

Notes: How do you feel about your eating today? Jot down your thoughts here.

_____

_____

TOP TEN SUPPLEMENTS

"Lack of energy" is one of the most common complaints that doctors hear from their patients. Supplements can help with energy and other problems. But they're no substitute for healthy food and they aren't going to help much if you eat poorly or rely on stimulants to cure fatigue, moodiness, or hunger.

The effects of herbal remedies, vitamins, and other supplements may be more subtle and gradual than the quick effects that come from taking a nonprescription pain reliever, snacking on something sugary, or drinking a cup of coffee. But supplements can help you along if you practice sensible eating, regular exercise, and a healthy lifestyle.

If you use supplements, never exceed the recommended dosage and always check with your physician to rule out adverse interactions with medications.

1. *A daily multivitamin* is important to your overall health. In 2003, a leading medical journal recommended that every American should take a multivitamin. Vitamins and minerals are like your body's checks and balances. Too many or too few can lead to health problems. In today's eat-and-run world, many of us are not getting the daily nutrients we need. In addition, our bodies change throughout every phase of our lives. Therefore, our needs for different vitamins and minerals change as well. We need vitamins like A, C, and E to serve as powerful antioxidants that fight free-radical damage caused by everyday stressors like pollution, smoking, high-fat diets, emotional upheaval, and even exercise. In essence, they protect the body from cell damage. The B vitamins have a codependent relationship, and they need each other to perform effectively. The body does not store them well so it's important to ingest them daily. The B vitamins are essential for energy production and keep the body's normal functions working. Anything from listening to loud music to losing your car keys can increase blood pressure and stress levels, causing the body to work less efficiently. Your daily multivitamin is insurance to maintain a solid nutritional foundation.

2. *L-carnitine* is an amino acid found in animal protein. It helps to metabolize fats and convert them into energy. L-carnitine has been shown to improve energy levels and may help with weight loss. It is available in pill form, or as part of a healthy diet that includes red meat. Over the past few years, L-carnitine has attracted increasing interest from athletes and sports enthusiasts as an aid for increasing energy and performance.

3. *Ginseng* has been used as a tonic in Chinese medicine for more than two thousand years. It has been shown to improve mood, alleviate stress, and improve mental and physical vitality. There are even indications that it can help fight cancer. It is commonly used to improve mental and physical vitality.

4. *Vitamin A* is one of my favorites. It's associated with immunity. And you don't have to take supplements to get your daily supply of vitamin A. Good food sources of beta-carotene, which in your body converts to vitamin A, are carrots, sweet potatoes, broccoli, spinach, and pumpkin. Vitamin A has also been shown to help prevent skin cancer. I make sure I eat lots of beta-carotene–rich foods for this reason.

5. *Vitamin C* is the beauty "drug." It helps maintain your skin, hair, and nails. It is one of the building blocks of collagen that keeps your skin looking firm and supple. Vitamin C protects the immune system and works as a powerful antioxidant. In addition to its supplement form, vitamin C comes in a variety of delicious flavors in fruits and vegetables such as oranges, berries, broccoli, and spinach.

6. *Soy* and its benefits have garnered hundreds of headlines in recent years. Soy is a form of protein and provides nutritional support for women before, during, and after the menopausal years. Getting more soy in your diet does not mean pouring soy sauce on your Chinese food! Try adding soy foods like tofu, soymilk, soy nuts, and soybeans (also known as edamame). Soy has been known for its cholesterol-lowering benefits. Try chocolate soymilk with a handful of almonds for a great snack. Try pouring soymilk over fresh berries for a delicious treat.

Order a large soy latte instead of one made with whole milk. You'll save about forty calories and about five grams of fat!

7. *Calcium* is another supplement I recommend, especially for aging women. Studies have linked insufficient calcium intake to osteoporosis. Calcium adds strength to your bones and teeth and plays an important role in other body functions. Recent studies have shown that calcium may help you lose weight. Calcium-rich foods include low-fat dairy and dark green leafy vegetables.

8. *Glucosamine and chondroitin* are components of natural joint cartilage. Preliminary research has shown that these supplements taken together can relieve joint pain, improve flexibility, and help slow the loss of cartilage associated with arthritis.

9. *"Probiotics"* is a term used to describe strains of beneficial bacteria, several of which are available in yogurt, that fight many of the organisms that cause illness in the digestive tract. These friendly bacteria help with digestive disorders that nobody likes to talk about, such as gas, bloating, and diarrhea. Some research has shown that probiotics are helpful in fighting colds and infections. Probiotics appear to assist the body's own natural defenses. Dietary sources of probiotics include sauerkraut, yogurt, sourdough bread, pickles, and cider vinegar. Supplements, including acidophilus and bifidobacteria, are available in capsule form. Use supplements for a few days whenever you complete a course of antibiotics to help restore your system's supply.

10. *Alfalfa* is an excellent source of vitamins, such as carotene, E, and K; minerals, such as potassium, calcium, and magnesium; eight amino acids; and chlorophyll. The leaves of this wonderful herb have natural diuretic and laxative properties. Practitioners of Chinese medicine have been using alfalfa since the sixth century to relieve fluid retention and swelling and as an overall health tonic. Alfalfa is available in tablet form.

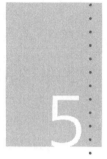

Feed Your Family, Feed Yourself

A child of five would understand this. Send someone to fetch a child of five.

—GROUCHO MARX

As parents, it's our job to worry about the health of our children. We try to make sure they're dressed warmly, we worry about them getting hurt, we spend whatever it costs to outfit them in helmets and pads for the sports they play, and we do our best to keep all their vaccinations up to date. But the biggest health problem facing our kids seems to lie somewhere between the television and the refrigerator. Childhood obesity in this country has become an epidemic.

- According to a study by the Kaiser Family Foundation in 2000, more than 15 percent of American children between the ages of six and eleven were overweight, up from only 4.2 percent in the 1960s.

- According to a 2001 study by the Lucile Packard Foundation for Children's Health, approximately one in four California fifth-, seventh-, and ninth-graders is overweight.

- According to the American Academy of Pediatrics, between 8 and 45 percent of newly diagnosed cases of childhood diabetes are type 2, the non-insulin-dependent variety of the disease, which is associated with obesity.

- According to the National Institutes of Health, childhood obesity increases the risk of health problems ranging from high blood pressure and high cholesterol to orthopedic problems, liver disease, and sleep apnea.

- A study released in the *Journal of the American Medical Association* found that the United States has the highest prevalence of overweight teens of the countries studied.

It's easy to blame fast food, supersized portions, television advertising, and sedentary pastimes like computer games. But it's harder to figure out what to do in the face of so much opposition. You can't monitor what your children put in their mouths every minute of the day. And laying down the law "because Mommy says so" only makes those forbidden treats more desirable.

MAKE IT A FAMILY AFFAIR

For me, the solution has been to get the whole family involved in the cause of healthy eating and obesity prevention. I teach my kids about the differences between healthy food choices and junk food. They know how protein works in their bodies, they know what carbohydrates are, they understand that partially hydrogenated oils are bad for them—and they know that most snack foods are loaded with them.

Because they're informed about food and nutrition, my kids are willing to try the healthier snack items that aren't made with partially hydrogenated oils. Some they like and some they don't. That's okay. They are learning how to think for themselves and decide what to eat and what not to eat. They are actually aware of how many treats they eat in a day. And they are reasonable when I say, "No more sugar," because they understand the facts.

Don't get me wrong: Our kitchen is not a perfect, pristine cornucopia of carrot sticks and wheat germ. I buy sugary cereals once in a while. Every so often, we have toaster pastries, doughnuts, and ice cream. But here's the key: I buy these foods occasionally. They are not staples—they are treats. They are exciting and fun, and my kids are always glad to see them. But we eat them in small portions.

We also count our five fruits and vegetables every day. We make sure we get in our protein, our calcium, and even our glasses of water.

They may not like everything at first, and I know that when they go to someone else's house or a party, they eat junk, and I'm okay with that. But they usually make good choices, and the best thing is that they are aware of how they feel when they eat too much junk. They actually now know when to stop because they don't like how they feel.

DOABLE DINNERS

I cook simply. Kids don't like complicated recipes with strange ingredients. Kids like it simple, so I cook chicken breasts, put some fresh fruit on the table, and add a salad or a steamed vegetable I know they like. (I season my veggies with kosher salt and balsamic vinegar, and the kids love it.) Occasionally I'll throw in some brown rice or baked potatoes. Or I'll make some sweet potatoes for my husband and myself.

In less than the time it would take to microwave enough frozen dinners for my family of five, I make healthy dinners with real food. Here are a few Freytag family favorites:

- I make tacos with ground turkey instead of ground beef. Add lettuce, tomatoes, and shredded cheese. Yum!

Family Food Chart

	Mom	Dad	Billy	Sally
Exercise				
M	*	*	*	*
T			*	*
W	*	*	*	*
T		*		*
F	*		*	
S	*	*	*	*
S				
Good food				
M	*	*	*	*
T	*	*		
W	*	*	*	
T			*	*
F	*		*	*
S				
S				

Charting Everyone's Progress

I'm a huge believer in using charts to keep a family on track. And I know that getting stars next to your name is a powerful motivator at any age! So I thought this chart, created by the American Council on Exercise, was a great idea for keeping the whole family focused on eating well and staying active.

Reprinted with permission from the American Council on Exercise. (www.acefitness.org)

- I put ground flaxseed in my spaghetti sauce (to add some healthy omega-3 oils to the meal) with some Parmesan cheese to disguise the flavor and serve it over whole-wheat pasta with some cubed chicken chunks or meatballs. Add some fruit and a glass of milk and you are set.

- I make hamburgers on my indoor grill with lean ground beef and serve them on whole-wheat buns with a slice of cheese, some pickles, and lettuce. Add cut-up fruit and some yogurt for the kids and make a fun salad for the grown-ups.

- We eat scrambled eggs for dinner with turkey sausage and fruit. Try making the eggs with skim milk, some onion and garlic powder, and a little fat-free cottage cheese. Blend them in the blender to make them fluffy and cook in a nonstick pan over medium heat until set.

And because we're a busy family, like everyone else, we will occasionally go to the drive-thru. I always remind the kids that it's a treat, but that it's full of fat and chemicals and will damage our insides if we eat it every day. But if we indulge occasionally, it's okay. We opt often for the healthier fast-food options. Many popular chains are offering nutritious alternatives like salads, wraps, and sandwiches that are lower in calories and fat than the traditional burgers and fried fare. Top with salsa for extra flavor.

SNACK STRATEGIES

If you've got the right stuff in your kitchen, it's just as easy to give your kids healthy snacks. I always have fresh fruit on hand, and we have a water cooler with paper cups in our kitchen. I make popcorn on the stove as a substitute for processed chips. I'll give them a piece of toast with light cinnamon sugar and some fruit or a bowl of cereal as a snack—the healthy kind, of course! Try carrots and celery, or apple slices dipped in peanut butter. My kids love peanuts. They also eat pretzels a lot. When I buy chips, they're the natural kind, made without partially hydrogenated oils. My kids have learned to like the cheese puffs and corn chips. I buy old-fashioned hard granola bars, not the chewy packaged snacks full of extra sugar and partially hydrogenated oils.

WILLS AND WON'TS

Here's the biggest thing: Parents need willpower to keep from giving in to their kids. My kids have been known to wheedle and whine to try and get me to give in—especially when they were toddlers. Now they know better, but still, even now, we can be driving home from an activity, and my kids will start in on the nagging. "Let's have McDonald's, please!" Sometimes I give in, but more often then not, I stand firm on eating at home, and by the time we get home, they've accepted it. After all, even peanut butter and jelly has more nutrition than most fast foods!

Believe me, I know how all that pleading can wear you down and how often the easiest thing to do is just give in to stop the whining. Don't do it: They will learn from the limits you set.

Kids actually like limits because subconsciously they make them feel safe. Your limits let your kids know you actually care!

Parents need to be active participants in their children's food choices. It's the best strategy for the long term. You don't have to shove it down their throats. Trying to exert too much control won't make your children confident about their abilities to choose wisely for themselves. Instead of trying to rule food with an iron fist, parents need to educate kids so they can make good decisions on their own. I don't deprive; I educate and help keep things in moderation!

The best way to deal with childhood obesity is to make it a family affair. When the entire family changes the behaviors that create the problem—poor eating habits and inactivity—the entire family benefits.

When well-meaning parents try to put their overweight children on special diets and exercise regimens that fall outside of the family routine, they usually only achieve minimal, short-term results. But when parents make healthy eating and being more physically active

Showdown in Aisle Five

Recently I was grocery shopping with my son and we were in the cereal aisle. All the free gifts and gimmicks in the boxes were catching his eye. He knows sugar cereals are a treat. So he'd grab one sugary brand after another from the shelf and ask, "Is this one healthy?" Of course, my answers were always "No." So he began to make a scene. All kids do this. Other moms passed us and gave me understanding looks. I could have given in. But I held my ground. I told him which ones he could choose. Then I told him I was leaving the aisle, and I rolled our cart around the corner. In a few seconds, he had followed me into the next aisle with a box of Raisin Bran.

I know how hard it is to reason with kids under five. But I tell parents all the time to hang in there: By the time their kids get to be seven, they will start to get it.

a family priority, and they don't single out their overweight children with special treatment, they give them the best possible chance to create healthy habits that will last them a lifetime.

And, frankly, these habits are good for you too. For instance, children should eat breakfast every day and take a daily multivitamin. So should you. And despite your crazy and busy schedules, you can try to have family dinners occasionally. You don't have to put on an apron and serve up a roast every night like June Cleaver, but you can have balanced nutrition and real food.

After all, it is very hard for a child to eat healthy and be active if other family members are eating potato chips and ice cream and watching a lot of TV! Everyone in the family can benefit from being more active and eating more fruits and vegetables and more low-fat dairy products.

The first step in developing a healthy family lifestyle is for parents to take a look in the mirror! Kids imitate and emulate their parents! Examine your own behavior and recognize how it influences your children. It does no good if your actions tell your child, "You can't sit around the house and eat potato chips, but I can."

You also need to take a close look at your home environment. Stocking the house with junk food and eating family meals in front of the television creates conditions conducive to weight problems. Taking daily walks with your kids, playing ball, and going to the park are great ways to add physical activity to a sedentary family schedule. And these activities help to reduce a child's time in front of the television and the computer, where, according to studies, the average child eats six hundred calories a day. If you can manage to cut that in half, it's worth five pounds a year!

Because no one wants to suffer from disease, I often explain to my kids what happens to their bodies when they have too much sugar, not enough nutrients, and too little exercise. Kids naturally don't want to be unhealthy or overweight. However, they don't do the grocery shopping, they usually don't decide the family meal, and they often don't even decide their portion sizes. But you do! By setting good examples, you all can benefit, you all can eat the same meal, and you all can be less stressed and feel better.

I use the Best-Better-Bad diet with my kids to teach them proper nutrition by linking foods to the choices. Low-calorie foods and "real foods" are "best" and can be eaten freely. Moderate-calorie foods, like pretzels, are "better" and can be eaten in moderation. High-calorie foods, like fast food, chips, crackers, sugar, and candy, are "bad" choices and should be eaten rarely and in small portions.

So it's not like it's no fun to eat at my house. We enjoy my home-made muffins but I promote them from "bad" to "better" by making them with a little flaxseed, trans fat–free margarine, and whole-wheat flour. And then we eat them in moderation.

THE 'TWEEN AND TEEN YEARS

The older your children are, the more challenging getting them to eat and live healthily can be. We all know that encouraging kids to exercise is not an easy task, because fitness competes with video games, movie rentals, computers, and 250 channels on cable television. The group of people called Generation Y were born between 1977 and 1994. This age group has a ravenous appetite for unhealthy dietary habits.

Generation Y is the largest population group since the baby boomers. They will be an important part of out country's future!

I hear a lot of parents say that even though these kids are over-indulging, they'll eventually outgrow the baby fat. But it isn't baby fat when they're thirteen. In the words of my kids: "Whatever!"

When it comes to older kids, setting a good example is even more important. If they spend these critical years without healthy role models, and without education about health and nutrition, they are starting a life-time of bad habits that will be even harder to break in adulthood.

Adolescence is a challenging time. They're faced with so many phys-ical, emotional, and social issues. These changes can often result in un-healthy and irregular eating behaviors such as skipping meals and cutting out food groups. (I recently watched a group of teenage girls at a party. They wouldn't eat the hamburgers being served be-cause they had all decided to become vegetarians. Instead, they were wolfing

I May Not Be Perfect but They Know I'm Trying

One day, I was driving with my daughter. I had just yelled at her about something. So I told her that I was sorry for losing my temper and that I shouldn't have been so upset. She replied, to make me feel better, "That's okay, Mom, you're really a good mom." And she reeled off a list of some projects I'd helped her with recently. At the end of her list of my good deeds was: "And you help me make healthy food choices!"

down red licorice by the pound.) Their eating habits may deteriorate to the point where they're indulging in late-night bingeing followed by fasting the next day. These dysfunctional eating behaviors are further aggravated by the sedentary yet busy lifestyles that have become the norm.

Even though today's teens are eating and drinking nearly twice as many calories as their parents did at their age, they may not be getting the nutrients they need to support growth. However, they are filling up on sugary sodas, candies, chips, fast food, and whatever else the food companies market to them. School cafeterias often make matters worse by offering junk food and vending machines in an attempt to cut costs and give kids what they want.

This is a unique time in human history. For the first time, society has too much. Yet we suffer from both too many calories and too few nutrients. What a strange problem! Malnourished used to mean scrawny. Now it could mean fat.

The struggle with food is especially hard on girls. Many young girls start their first diet in junior high school in an attempt to attain that perfect, air-brushed, digitally altered magazine image. So kids don't have any energy, yet they're overweight. The pressure to be thin amidst the constant marketing of junk food creates stress and potential eating disorders. Insufficient levels of nutrients can also affect the balance of hormones in children as they grow.

The big issue is that kids are inundated with the images of the thin, the beautiful, and the fashionable. Yet the same media outlets that put forth these images also entice them with a nonstop array of fast-food advertising, where products loaded with fat and calories are made to look delicious, fun, and cool.

So fitness is especially important for older children and teens. Unfortunately, due to funding problems, many schools have no physical education. As a result, Generation Y is turning into Generation XL, with decades of disastrous health consequences yet to come.

My message is, let's teach these kids life skills and give them the knowledge and the opportunity to form good habits that will carry them into adulthood. Fitness and nutrition need to be skills that we teach them along with how to drive a car and how to live on a budget.

Equip your kids with the knowledge they need to read nutrition la-

Top Tips for Busy Families

1. Keep your kitchen stocked with healthy convenience foods like fresh fruit, frozen veggies, chicken breasts, brown rice, fresh eggs, and whole-grain pastas.

2. Encourage your kids to drink water—and like it. Try keeping bottles of lightly flavored water in the fridge instead of soda pop.

3. Make Sunday your cooking day. Prepare a soup that can be served a couple of times during the week. Or make extra spaghetti sauce to freeze. Cook chicken breasts so that they're ready to go for salads and sandwiches.

4. Get into a good rut! If your family likes a particular meal, there's no rule that says you can't rely on it every week. When I was growing up, every Saturday was hamburger night and every Sunday was soup and sandwich night. Nothing wrong with that.

5. Get your kids involved. Older kids can help cook. Even younger kids will appreciate being asked to help with planning and grocery shopping.

6. Take fifteen minutes once a week to plan your meals before you go to the grocery store. You'll definitely save more time than you spend. Imagine how much time you'd have for other things if you only went to the store once a week!

7. Get a head start on side dishes. Prepare a double recipe of one versatile side dish, like sweet potatoes or rice, which can be reheated later in the week.

8. Meet them halfway. If you suspect that your kids will rebel if you serve them a plateful of brown rice or whole-wheat spaghetti, try mixing half of the whole grain with half of the more familiar, refined product. Eventually, you might be able to phase the refined stuff out altogether.

9. Don't use sweets to bribe or reward. Fruits and vegetables taste sweeter to kids whose palates aren't used to sugar.

10. Upgrade your own eating. If you learn to enjoy eating well, your children will too!

bels and make informed decisions about how much is too much and how much is not enough. Kids are smart. They can figure it out. Let's face it, their memories are often better than ours! When kids understand the potential risks for their health, they will often choose to make healthier decisions based on logic.

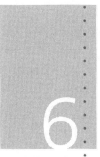

Moving Parts:
The Importance of Exercise

Success is the sum of small efforts, repeated day in and day out.

ROBERT J. COLLIER (1876–1918), WRITER

Why should you exercise? After all, you don't need to be physically fit to survive in modern society. We don't have to hunt and grow and gather our own food anymore. And there are so many other things to do—like holding on to our jobs, paying our bills, and looking after our families.

You probably know exercise is good for you. But you probably don't know where you'll fit it into your day. And you can expend an enormous amount of energy figuring out why you can't find time to exercise:

"I can't exercise in the morning because I'm not a morning person."

"I can't exercise during my lunch hour because I don't want to be sweaty."

"I can't exercise when I get home from work because I have to fix dinner."

"I can't exercise in the evening because I'm too tired."

"I can't exercise because I'm too out of shape."

Unfortunately all that energy burned is mental energy. It doesn't actually burn any calories. And that's what losing body fat is on a fundamental level: calories in versus calories out. It's simple math: You need to expend more calories per day than you take in.

Exercise offers you other benefits besides burning calories. As we age, our bodies start to change. We gradually lose muscle strength, so we can't lift and carry as much as we used to. We lose flexibility, diminishing our range of motion, so we can't reach and bend as far as we used to. The loss of muscle strength and flexibility makes our joints more vulnerable to injury and strain, so we feel more aches and pains when we do yard work and play outside with our kids.

There are even more long-term benefits to regular exercise. It can reduce cholesterol levels, decrease blood pressure, and make your heart more efficient. Exercising can even increase your life expectancy! A recent study showed that people who are overweight at forty are likely to die at least three years sooner than those who are slim. In other words, being fat during middle age can be just as dangerous as smoking.

Regular exercise can slow down the aging process and even reverse it to a degree. Americans are obsessed with staying young and the most reliable, most affordable way to do it is to exercise and eat well. Vibrant, glowing good health is one luxury you can't buy. Moving your body every day is a bargain compared with all the face creams and cellulite creams money can buy. And it's an even bigger bargain compared to the alternative. You can't buy a healthy heart—but you can earn it.

More than half of all American adults get little or no exercise according to the Centers for Disease Control and Prevention. To people who are busy, stressed, and overcommitted, the primary drawback to exercise is that it takes up time—and that's the one thing most of us don't have. When you invest your time in exercise, that investment pays you back generously, giving you extra energy to help you cope with your busy life, better health to help you manage your stress, and greater confidence to help you meet your challenges head-on.

It may not be easy for you to find the time. But your dream of a better body can't come true unless you do. If you have a demanding job and little kids, you'll need to be creative. Maybe you can ask your spouse or neighbor to watch your kids while you work out. Maybe you can set your alarm a little earlier in the morning. Studies show that "I'll do it later" usually turns into never. That's why I'm a proponent of morning exercise. While it might be tough to get up earlier at first, getting regular exercise will help you sleep better—which will help you wake up easier in the mornings.

If you're trying to find time to get moving, one of the first places to look is right in front of your television. If you spend thirty minutes a day watching your favorite programs, think about using that time to move your body. With the right home-exercise equipment, you don't even have to miss a minute of the shows you really like.

THE FOUR ELEMENTS OF A HEALTHY EXERCISE REGIMEN

Maybe you've tried walking or swimming or other kinds of exercise in the past but you've been disappointed by the results—you didn't lose the weight you wanted to lose or you didn't look as good as you'd hoped. That's because your body needs more than one type of exercise. For an optimal exercise program, you need to incorporate all of the following types of exercise into your regimen.

Cardio Exercise

Jogging, swimming, and brisk walking are all cardiovascular workouts, meaning they all improve the health of your heart (cardio) and circulatory system (vascular). When you perform cardio exercise, your heart beats faster and you breathe a little harder. The cardio equipment you'll find at a health club—like elliptical trainers, stationary bikes, step machines, rowing machines, and treadmills—are all designed to accomplish the same thing.

Cardio workouts are important for weight loss because these activities burn more calories than other kinds of exercise. Cardio fitness also makes you less vulnerable to heart disease and clogged arteries. Weight-bearing cardio exercise (like walking, jogging, and jumping rope) can also help you maintain bone density, which can prevent osteoporosis, a real-life concern for women as we age.

The best-case cardio regimen for weight loss is at least thirty minutes of cardio exercise per day, three to five days a week. If you can't fit a thirty-minute workout into your schedule, you can do two fifteen-minute work-outs or even three ten-minute workouts.

Sometimes your life will be so crazy and your schedule will be so hectic, you won't be able to find thirty minutes. Don't give up. Remember: All movement is good movement. Ten minutes is always better than nothing. Three times a week is always better than zero times a week. The cardio workouts in chapter 7 are designed to give you the variety and adaptability you need to get your heart pumping faster no matter what's on your calendar.

Strength Training

The terms "strength training" and "resistance training" are used interchangeably to refer to exercise that builds muscle. Lifting weights is one example of strength training. Using resistance bands is another example. Some strength exercises don't need any equipment at all—push-ups, squats, and lunges all use the weight of your own body to provide the necessary resistance for your muscles to exert against.

Strength training has been one of the biggest exercise trends in the last decade—and for good reason. Muscles burn more calories, whether you're jogging on the treadmill or napping on the couch. We tend to lose muscle mass as we age and this muscle loss slows down our metabolism. This may be why you're gaining weight even though you aren't eating any more than you used to. With a lower percentage of muscle, your body is burning fewer calories a day.

Strength training also makes it easier for your body to handle the physical stresses of the typical day. Strong arms and shoulders help you lift your groceries and carry your kids around. Stronger leg muscles protect your knee and ankle joints when you're climbing stairs or running to catch a bus. Studies have also shown that strength training is even more important than cardio in helping to prevent osteoporosis.

However, the real reason most people are taking up strength training is that toned muscle makes you look better. A pound of muscle takes up 14 percent less space than a pound of fat. That means you'll look slimmer and your clothes will be looser, even if the scale doesn't budge.

To build muscle and rev your metabolism, aim for two to three strength-training sessions per week, using the strength workouts in chapter 8.

You can do full-body strength training two or three days a week. Or, if you are pressed for time, do a little strength training every day. If you are sore, allow twenty-four to forty-eight hours between strength workouts to give your muscles a chance to rest and rebuild.

Core Training

When trainers talk about your "core" or your "powerhouse," they're talking about the muscles in your abdomen, back, and sides. These are the muscles that you don't often think about until they hurt, but you use them all the time—standing, sitting, and even lying down. Your core supports your spine and protects your back from strain and injury. When these muscles are strong and toned, you stand up straighter. Your tummy gets flatter and your waist looks smaller. A well-toned torso makes your whole body look—and feel—slimmer, fitter, and healthier.

Many of the most popular core exercises practiced today are inspired by the Pilates method. Almost a century ago, a German man named Joseph Pilates created a system of strengthening and stretching exercises to help his own body recover and rebuild after an illness. He brought his system to the United States in the 1920s. For decades, the Pilates method was a well-kept secret among athletes and dancers who needed to develop and maintain a strong, lean musculature. Within the last couple of decades, as the Pilates method has become more widely known, exercise physiologists and trainers have expanded upon the principles of Joseph Pilates. Today an emphasis on core training is an integral part of any fitness plan.

You'll notice that improving your core strength will have a positive impact on every move you make. You'll sit up straighter, walk with more confidence, and handle physical stresses of all kinds with greater ease. Aim for two to three core sessions per week, using the core workout in chapter 9.

Stretching

Flexibility is something that you don't appreciate until you start to lose it. As long as I can remember, fitness experts have endorsed stretching as an integral part of any fitness program. Stretching minimizes your risk of injury, relieves the pain and discomfort of stiff muscles, and improves athletic performance.

Top Stress-Busting Benefits of Exercise 10

Study after study has shown that regular exercise makes you feel good. Even when your kids are cranky and your boss is moody and your spouse is sulky, you can always count on the physical and mental uplift you can generate just by getting your heart pumping and your muscles moving. Stress actually causes you to breathe more shallowly, depriving your body of oxygen just when you need it most. A good brisk walk practically forces you to breathe. Plus you don't need a prescription and there are no side effects.

1. It alleviates anxiety. Studies show that people feel less nervous and more relaxed after they exercise.

2. It can lighten depression. Chronic stress can wear you down and leave you feeling hopeless. Movement therapy is often used to treat depression patients. Remember: Any movement is good movement!

3. It can help you sleep like a baby. If your worries are keeping you awake, you'll be even less prepared to deal with them in the morning. I always liken this phenomenon to parents trying to tire their kids out so that they'll sleep well. That's exactly what you want to do: tire yourself out. If we don't move, we bottle up that energy inside us. Numerous studies have shown that regular exercisers enjoy better sleep.

4. This may seem contradictory, but it can also boost your energy. Energy is like money: Just like you have to spend money to make money, you've got to expend energy to make energy. Stress depletes your reserves and resources but exercise will always restore you.

5. It's a mood booster. When you perform cardio exercise, endorphins are released into your bloodstream. Endorphins, chemicals produced in the brain, make you feel good, even euphoric. These natural "happy drugs" are responsible for decreasing feelings of pain and stress. Just one workout will elevate your mood and leave you with a feeling of well-being that lasts up to two hours after your workout ends.

6. It makes you more alert. As your muscles contract and relax, your brain responds by releasing certain neurotransmitters, the brain chemicals that carry messages between nerve cells and muscles. These promote both relaxation and alertness.

7. It enhances self-esteem by giving you a positive feeling of accomplishment. When your inner critic starts telling you that you aren't coping well, silence that nagging little voice by reviewing your accomplishments in your workout log!

8. It helps you flush the by-products of stress out of your system. Stressful episodes cause hormones like adrenaline to be released into your bloodstream. Vigorous activity helps your body wipe the slate clean.

9. It inspires you to be a healthier eater. Once you start feeling like an athlete, you'll start eating like one. You'll start thinking of food as fuel for your engine. You'll be more aware of how your body feels when you try to take out your troubles on a pizza. The better nourished you are, the better able you are to cope with stress.

10. It reminds you to take care of yourself. Before you can give anything to anyone, you've got to be kind and generous to yourself first.

You should stretch after your workout to cool down the body when muscles are warmed from the blood-pumping effects of exercise. The aims of stretching are to gently lengthen muscles, maintain tissue elasticity, and encourage flexibility. You'll notice that regular stretching will increase the range of motion in your joints, making it easier to move through your everyday tasks.

Most of the flexibility moves I recommend come from yoga, a fitness tradition from India that has been practiced for centuries. The gentle, deliberate moves of yoga teach you to tune into your body and pay attention to your posture, breathing, and alignment. The flexibility workout in chapter 10 will introduce you to some fundamental yoga poses that will help to keep you limber for a lifetime.

CREATING A HOME GYM

Stocking your home with a few well-chosen pieces of exercise gear can be a real advantage as you're trying to start and maintain a consistent fitness regimen. Having your own gear handy puts you in control. It saves you time, since you never have to drive to and from the health club. It gives you a weatherproof alternative to outdoor activities like walking or biking. And it lets you squeeze in exercise on your own timetable. You can work out in the morning before the kids wake up or in the evening while you're watching your favorite television program. Even if you have a gym membership, home equipment is a lifesaver for those days when you just don't have time to get there.

Here are the basics. Of course the choices are up to you, depending on what you'll enjoy using, what you can afford, and what you have room for. Resist the temptation to pick up a few random items on sale; if the item is poorly constructed or doesn't really interest you, it's not a bargain.

- *Balance ball* Also known as a stability ball. You can use this ball by itself for abdominal crunches and stretches or use it in conjunction with hand weights as a substitute for a weight bench. When you sit on or lie across the balance ball, you engage all the muscles in your core to keep yourself balanced.

- *Bosu Ball®* This device looks like a balance ball cut in half. It's much safer to stand on than a balance ball. This ball is designed to improve your balance and stability for exercises performed in both sitting and standing positions.

- *Cardio equipment* People always ask me which cardio machine burns the most calories. And I always say: It's the one you'll use the most! The more you like it, the longer you'll stay on it. And the longer you stay on it, the more calories you'll burn! If you have the space and the budget, you can choose from a variety of treadmills, exercise bikes, and elliptical trainers.

  Thanks to technological advances, there are lots of affordable options; you can find good, high-quality cardio equipment as low as $300 up to $1000 depending on the extra features. And these machines are designed for your home—you can find treadmills that fold and elliptical trainers that wheel away for storage. Treadmills continue to be the most purchased cardio equipment because walking is America's favorite form of exercise.

- *Hand weights* Also known as dumbbells. Weights are great for building

Susie T., pictured below, lost eighteen pounds in sixty days and went down two dress sizes by using the Motivating Bodies lifestyle plan.

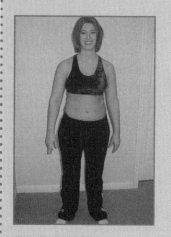

6.1 • Susie (before)

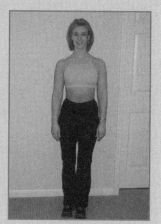

6.2 • Susie (after)

muscle and sculpting your body. One pair each of two-, three-, and five-pound weights will be enough to get you going on a beginning strength-training regimen. Add eight- and ten-pound weights as your strength improves.

- *Pedometer* Accumulating between four thousand and six thousand steps per day puts you in line with most recommendations for thirty minutes of physical activity daily. However, for weight loss, I recommend gradually working toward a goal of ten thousand steps per day; that's about five miles' worth of walking. Two thousand steps is approximately one mile. Every step counts, whether you're tidying up your house, shopping for groceries, or walking the dog. Counting your steps with a pedometer is a great way to see how active you really are. The pedometer is a great mental game and a great motivator. When you wear one, you can't help checking it to see how you're doing!

- *Resistance bands* Like hand weights, these items help you build muscle by providing resistance. Unlike weights, they're easy to store and handy for traveling.

- *VCR or DVD player* If you like taking exercise classes but you can't make it to the gym, having a couple of workouts on video or DVD can add fun and variety to your regimen. Exercise tapes are also a fun way to get your kids involved. Kids love to join in. It's great family time.

- *Yoga mat* Also known as a sticky mat. The surface isn't really sticky; it's just a rubbery, nonslip material that makes it easier, safer, and more comfortable to do yoga and other stretching exercises.

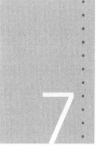

The Heart of the Matter:
Cardiovascular Exercise

It is hard to fail but it is worse never to have tried to succeed.

—THEODORE ROOSEVELT

Our bodies were built for motion. We weren't designed to spend all our waking hours slumped in front of a computer and stuck behind the wheel of a car. Motion is basic human nature. As soon as toddlers are old enough to move around on their own two feet, they start running all over the place—and they don't stop until they get old enough to be mesmerized by television and computer games.

For many of us, once we stop being kids, it's very hard to get moving again. We've forgotten how good it feels to fly across the backyard as fast as our feet can carry us. As adults, we can recapture that joy. But first I want you to simply get used to moving your body again. Cardio exercise is motion at its most basic. You swing your arms, you pump your legs, and, in doing so, you burn calories.

Shedding that body fat is easy math. It's calories in minus calories out. How can you do this without severe dieting? It's easy: take full, deep breaths; get the heart pumping; and get your body in motion!

If you are just getting started, keep it simple and don't psych yourself out. Start with baby steps and move up to workouts with more difficulty and length. If you are already a moderately active exerciser, you can challenge yourself with something more intense.

Try to get in a cardio workout three to five days a week. Start slowly at first. If you've been very sedentary or are significantly overweight, you may only be able to manage a few minutes a day at first. Don't get discouraged if you can't do as much as you want at first. Something is always better than nothing. You have to start somewhere. Don't underestimate the importance of whatever you manage to do. As long as you get yourself going, you've made valuable progress toward a very important goal. As Ally McBeal once said: "You can't win the raffle if you don't buy the ticket."

WINNING THE RATINGS GAME

In the following cardio workouts, I'll refer to various RPE numbers. Trainers and exercise physiologists use the rate of perceived exertion (RPE) scale to measure the amount of effort you feel as you're exercising. It's a great way to get in touch with how hard you are working.

The RPE scale also teaches you that you're in charge of your body—it's your interpretation of how you're feeling, not your high-school gym teacher's insistence on how you should be feeling.

RPE Scale	
0 – 1	Little to no exertion; you're lying on the couch, lifting nothing heavier than a potato chip.
2 – 3	You're moving, but it's easy and slow, just stretching and strolling; this is how you warm up your body before exercise and cool down afterward.
4 – 5	Your muscles are warm and you're starting to sweat; your breathing rate is slightly elevated but you can still hold a conversation.
6 – 7	You're working harder but you can still take a sip from your water bottle and utter a full sentence without gasping.
8 – 9	You're breathing hard and getting close to your limit; you can only say a few words.
10	This is the absolute limit of what you can do; you can't waste a breath on a single word.

Getting good, effective cardio exercise doesn't mean you have to spend half an hour gasping for air at an RPE of 9. Throw that tired, old "no pain, no gain" slogan out the window. Exercise should not be painful. If riding a bike or using an elliptical trainer is uncomfortable, try lowering the resistance. Maybe you need to start with a walking program and then add the hills on your treadmill. Honor your body and listen to what it's saying to you.

YOUR TARGET HEART RATE

Another way to determine effort is to monitor your heart rate while working out. The target heart rate is a range of beats per minute where your body is working hard enough to reap the benefits of cardio exercise but not so hard as to risk injury. Your age and fitness level determine your target heart rate. Remember that your target heart rate is just a guide, so listen to your body for indications of pain or overexertion. Here's the simplest way to calculate your target heart rate:

1. Subtract your age from 220. This is your maximum heart rate (MHR) in beats per minute.

2. Calculate 65 percent of your maximum rate. This is the low end of your target heart rate range.

3. The high end of the range is 85 percent of your maximum heart rate.

Let's use a forty-year-old exerciser as an example:

1. For our sample exerciser, the maximum heart rate calculation would look like this: $220 - 40 = 180$

2. For the low end of the target heart rate range, the math goes like this: $180 \times 0.65 = 117$.

3. $180 \times 0.85 = 153$.

So, a forty-year-old exerciser should try to keep her heart rate between 117 and 153 beats per minute. Many cardio machines have heart rate monitors built in. But you don't have to be tied to a machine. If your favorite form of cardio is walking or riding your bike outdoors, a heart rate monitor can go wherever you do. If you don't have a monitor, I recommend using the rate of perceived exertion (page 86) instead of trying to monitor your pulse by hand.

IT ALL ADDS UP

My latest exercise slogan is "every little effort counts." The harsh reality is that you have to burn a lot of calories to lose weight. So many exercisers overdo it at first. If you are overweight, you will find it hard to maintain a fast-paced workout for long periods of time. A better approach would be to burn calories by working out at a moderate pace several times a day. Consistency is more important than intensity when you are starting to exercise. To begin, be consistent each day. Then increase the exertion level of your workout gradually over the course of several weeks.

Here are some ideas to help you fit cardio into your life:

- Walk on your treadmill during television commercials. You'll get fifteen minutes of exercise in a one-hour program. If you have been exercising for a while and have built up endurance, walk during the program and take breaks during the commercials for forty-five minutes of exercise.

- Break it up. Ten minutes of exercise during the *Today* show plus ten minutes more during the *Tonight Show* equals twenty minutes.

- Get up early. I know it won't be easy at first, but a morning workout will make you feel good—physically and mentally—throughout the day. And those good feelings will help reinforce your morning workout habit.

THE MOTIVATING BODIES MOVE TO LOSE CARDIO PROGRAM

The basis of this cardio program is a walking workout that can be done outdoors or indoors on a treadmill. You can easily adapt these ideas to your bike or elliptical machine by using different resistance levels. The following workouts give you cardio choices for the workout schedule in chapter 11.

Option 1: The Essential Cardio Workout (Walk or Run)

Goal: Thirty minutes a day (including warm-up and cool-down).

Warm-up: Five minutes. Start by moving your body at a relaxed, easygoing pace. The purpose of a warm-up is to elevate your core body temperature and increase blood flow throughout your body, preparing your muscles and circulatory system for the work yet to come. Your heart rate should be no higher than 50 percent of your MHR. You're not trying to burn tons of calories here, but that doesn't mean you should skip it. You need to warm your muscles, lubricate your joints, and prepare for increased range of motion.

Contrary to popular belief, static stretching (holding a stretch for a long period of time) is not the way to go before exercise. It won't help reduce injury or prevent a pulled muscle. Stretching a cold muscle can even cause injury. Static stretching is best done after your workout when your muscles are warm and need to be lengthened.

Cardio: Twenty minutes. Try to maintain a fairly steady pace. Ideally, once you are warmed up, you can pick up the pace without causing strain or pain. If you're on a treadmill, aim to maintain a speed of three to five miles per hour (mph) or 65 to 85 percent of your MHR. Use the ranges below to determine the speed and heart rate that's right for you.

- Beginning walkers: 2.5 to 3.5 mph, or 65 percent MHR*

- Intermediate walkers: 3.5 to 4.0 mph, or 75 percent MHR*

- Advanced walkers or joggers: 4.0 to 4.5 mph brisk walk, above 4.5 mph light jog, or 85 percent MHR*

Cool-down: Five minutes. End your workout by slowing down your pace and breathing deeply. Let your heart rate recover a little and let your body cool off.

---

* These are suggestions, not musts. If you can't maintain these speeds or heart rates, it's no big deal. Just do as much as you can. Remember, every journey starts with the first step! If your first step is three minutes a day, it's still a good first step. If you can't do thirty minutes, do ten. And you'll still be able to measure your progress as you become more fit. If you are consistent, your endurance and capability will improve. Be patient and persistent. Try each day to go a little longer and a little farther. Eventually, you'll be able to work your way up to complete the essential workout. And you'll be amazed by the strength and confidence you'll gain. We are all in this together. I'm your biggest fan and commend you for taking each step!

Option 2: The Motivators Interval Workout

Goal: Thirty minutes a day (including warm-up and cool-down)

Warm-up: Five minutes.

Cardio: Twenty minutes. Pick up the pace from your warm-up and get ready to alternate between high intensity and low intensity, or recovery pace. Start with one-minute intervals: Do a minute of high intensity walking or jogging. You should be at about 7 to 8 on the RPE; you'll be breathing heavily through your mouth but still able to talk. Then slow down for a minute, working out at a 4 or 5 on the rate of perceived exertion scale (or at 40 to 50 percent MHR) to give your body a chance to recover. Alternate hard minutes with easy minutes for twenty minutes.

If you're on a treadmill, you can use the speed of the machine to create variations in intensity. Alternate intervals where you're walking at a brisk 4.0 or faster mph with recovery intervals at 3.0 mph.

As you become more fit, go for intervals that are two minutes long so that you're working hard for two minutes and then recovering for two minutes. Once the two-minute intervals start to feel easier, try three- or four-minute intervals.

Better yet, as you feel stronger, make your high-intensity intervals longer than your recovery intervals. Alternate four minutes of high intensity with two minutes of working at a recovery pace. If you're walking outdoors, use a stopwatch or a watch with a second hand to measure your intervals.

Increasing your speed isn't the only way to increase intensity. You can also challenge your body by adding hills to your outdoor walking route. On your treadmill, increase the incline. If you're using an exercise bike or elliptical trainer, you can simply increase the level of resistance.

Cool-down: Five minutes. End by

A Sore Subject

Injuries happen to everyone, from weekend warriors to experienced fitness professionals. If you take injuries seriously and give them the proper attention, they don't have to be major parking spots on your road to fitness. If you get shin splints or a pulled muscle, use the time-honored R.I.C.E. method:

- **R**est. The amount of time will vary with the severity of your injury. A pulled muscle will probably heal in a day or two. A sprained ankle may take a couple of weeks.

- **I**ce. Apply several times a day, for about twenty minutes at a time, for as long as pain persists. For best results, begin as soon as possible after the injury occurs.

- **C**ompress. If possible, wrap the injury firmly with an elastic bandage, taking care not to cut off circulation.

- **E**levate. When possible, keep the injury elevated to help reduce swelling.

Apply the R.I.C.E. method according to your own judgment. If pain, swelling, or stiffness persist beyond a day or two, call your doctor's office.

slowing down to an easy, comfortable pace and breathing deeply. Let your heart rate recover a little and let your body cool off.

Option 3: The Triple Cardio Workout (This is my favorite!)
Goal: Thirty minutes a day (including warm-up and cool-down).

Warm-up: Three to five minutes of your first activity. For example, if you're going to start with walking, walk slowly.

Cardio: Combine three different ten-minute activities to create a thirty-minute cross-training blast! This includes your warm-up and cool-down.

Here's an example for outdoors: Warm up by walking slowly for three minutes, then walk seven minutes at a moderate pace. Next, hop on your bike and do a quick ten-minute ride through the neighborhood. Then switch to your in-line skates, go about five minutes, and turn around to come home, slowing your pace down for the last three minutes. If you have access to a pool, you can substitute ten minutes of lap swimming for one of the activities.

Here's an example for the gym: Start with three minutes of walking slowly followed by seven minutes of walking briskly on the treadmill. Next, switch to the elliptical trainer and go for ten minutes. Then hop onto a bike or stair stepper and go for seven minutes at a brisk pace. Then slow down the machine for the remaining three minutes.

The triple workout helps time fly so it's a great antidote to boredom. And you will definitely feel it when you're done! Switching activities helps to tone many more muscles than a single-activity workout. It also challenges your heart and keeps you mentally engaged. There's nothing like a triple cardio workout to make you feel like a real cross-training athlete! Remember to use your RPE or monitor your heart rate to stay in that 65 to 85 percent of MHR zone.

Cool-down: Three to five minutes. Always use the last few minutes of your third activity to slow down. End by slowing down to an easy, comfortable pace and breathing deeply. Let your heart rate recover a little and let your body cool off.

How Healthy Are You?

1. Do you do cardio workouts at least four times a week?

2. Do you strength train two or three times a week?

3. Are you a nonsmoker?

4. Do you wear sunscreen?

5. Do you get at least seven hours of sleep a night?

6. Do you take a multivitamin every day?

7. Do you eat fresh or frozen fruits and veggies each day?

8. Do you eat fish or chicken each week?

9. Do you take a few minutes to meditate each day?

10. Do you drink no more than two cups of coffee each day?

11. Do you wear proper footwear and clothing so that you're safe and comfortable while you're exercising?

12. Do you own—and use regularly—any resistance bands or a stability ball?

See page 93 for scoring.

SAFETY MATTERS

Even though you're not jumping off your sofa to run a marathon, you still need to take precautions to safeguard your health and prevent injuries.

- Check with your doctor first. You need to know how much exertion your heart and joints can withstand. This is especially important the older you are, and the more overweight you are.

- Wear the appropriate clothes and shoes. Clothes that are too loose can trip you up or get caught on things. Clothes that are too tight can interfere with your circulation. If you're walking early in the morning or after dark, make sure drivers can see you by wearing light colors and reflective gear. Invest in the best pair of walking/running shoes you can afford.

- Start slowly. It's okay to be conservative at first, to give your body time to get used to movement. Don't pound yourself into the ground because you're in a hurry to see results or because you want to punish yourself for letting yourself go.

- Warm up with five minutes of gentle movement to help your body make the transition from stillness to motion.

- Remember to breathe! Your body needs more oxygen when you're working out.

- Stay hydrated. Replenish yourself by drinking four to six ounces of water for every fifteen minutes of exercise. I have a belt pack that holds a water bottle for hiking, biking, and jogging.

I always say, if you don't take the time to take care of yourself now, you may need to take even more time later.

POINTS OF INTEREST

The best way to keep yourself in the game is to make it *fun*. If you think of your workout as a chore, it will be a chore. If you think of it as your playtime, it will be something you look forward to. I always joke in fitness classes that the worst part is the first five minutes and the best part is walking out the door at the end. So remind yourself of how great it feels to finish a workout. Make that feeling your destination as you're lacing up your walking shoes or driving to the gym.

There are lots of ways to make fitness fun:

- Listen to music. I've even learned how to download songs onto my iPod or onto CDs. I program a series of "walk songs," alternating with "run songs" for my interval workout!

- Recruit a buddy. Exercising with friends adds the fun of lively conversation to the experience. And the buddy system helps you maintain consistency too. Breaking a workout promise you've made to yourself is much easier than standing up a friend who's waiting for you.

- Create several road maps to keep yourself interested and engaged. If you're walking or biking outdoors, don't stick to the same route day in and day out. Go left where you usually went right. Drive to a park and walk around a lake. If you are an outdoors person, have a few different trails or paths. If you're working out indoors, don't stare at the television all the time. Read the paper or browse through your favorite fashion magazine. Watch a movie: I'll watch half a movie while I'm on my treadmill, then save the second half for my next workout. Wanting to know how it ends becomes my motivation!

- If you're really pressed for time, you can even talk on the phone. Call up a friend who won't mistake you for a heavy breather. It's multitasking at its finest!

- Play mind games with yourself. If you're a parent of young children, you already know the drill. Tell yourself you only need to stay on the treadmill for five minutes. Or tell yourself you can quit after half a mile.

- Use a pedometer to tally up all your steps per day.

Scoring:

0–4 "Yes" answers: You should probably lie down to recover from taking this quiz!

5–6 "Yes" answers: Get a personal trainer pronto and put your doctor on speed dial!

7–9 "Yes" answers: You're pretty typical—but are you willing to settle for that?

10–11 "Yes" answers: Very good! Now, about those "No" answers . . .

12 "Yes" answers: You are a shining example of health and fitness!

FORM AND FUNCTION

As long as you're taking the time to move your body, you might as well make the most of it. Check in with yourself every few minutes to see if you're slumping or getting sloppy. If you carry yourself like an athlete, you feel like an athlete. You are an athlete.

- Stand tall when performing your cardio; keep your chest up and swing your arms naturally. Don't hunch over in the shoulder or hold tension in the neck. Relax the upper body.
- Hold your abs tight to protect your lower back.
- Pay attention to your body. Never work through pain. Learn to differentiate between pain and muscle fatigue. Pain is "Ouch, that hurts!" Muscle fatigue is "Wow, my muscles are tired; I can only go a little farther."

A CLASS ACT

Once you've been exercising for a few weeks, and you and your confidence are in better shape, think about attending an exercise class at a local health club or community center. Group fitness is a great way to stay on track and add variety to your workout.

I've been teaching and enjoying aerobic classes for fifteen years. Believe me, there have been plenty of days when I didn't feel like getting myself going, much less anyone else. But as soon as I walk into the studio, the energy of my students gives me a boost and I feel great by the end of the workout!

Taking a class offers novice exercisers several important advantages. You have an instructor who can teach you new moves. You'll be in the presence of other class members so you can see that you're not the only person in the world who is carrying around a few extra pounds. And, as you get to know the people in your class, they'll start to miss you if you don't show up—and you'll start to miss them!

Strong Language: *Strength Training*

8

Nothing great was ever achieved without enthusiasm.

—RALPH WALDO EMERSON

Ever since childhood I've been into weightlifting. It's not that I was playing around with dumbbells as a little kid, but I was active, pulling myself up in trees, playing ball, and doing the bent arm hang in gym class.

As an adult, I became passionate about weight training and I have spent years exploring a variety of body-sculpting and weight-training workouts. The advantages of weight training are numerous. As you age, weight training helps you to maintain your metabolism; keep your bones healthy; and improve your body's strength, power, endurance, and lean body tissue. Studies have shown that weight training offers mental benefits as well, boosting confidence and even alleviating depression.

My approach to weight training has become more moderate over the years, as my life has gotten busier. Yet I can't see myself ever doing without some sort of strength-training program.

With a little effort, strength training can make a dramatic difference in how you look and feel. If you're consistent, you can even achieve noticeable results in as little as ten minutes a day.

All too often, people who are trying to lose weight focus on cardio and forget (or perhaps don't know) how lifting weights can help them look slimmer and burn more calories all day long.

Your body uses the largest percentage of its daily caloric needs to maintain your resting metabolic rate (RMR). Your RMR is the number of calories you need at rest to maintain all of your body's vital processes and systems—digestion, breathing, circulation, tissue repair, and organ function. Lifting weights increases your muscle mass so you're not only burning calories while you're exercising, you're burning more calories while you're watching television and sleeping! The more muscle tissue you have, the more calories you burn. Each pound of muscle burns approximately thirty to fifty more calories per day at rest than a pound of body fat.

GETTING STARTED ON STRENGTH TRAINING

Although you can certainly do these weight routines at the gym, I've designed these workouts for the home exerciser. All you need is an exercise ball, a mat, and a few sets of hand weights or dumbbells. If you intend to use hand weights at home, plan on purchasing several different pairs in a variety of weights. Experiment to see which weights work for your level. Certain muscle groups like your chest and arms may be able to take more weight than smaller muscles like those in your shoulders.

The workouts in this chapter call for an exercise ball, also known as a stability ball. This is a large, lightweight, inflatable ball that you can sit on or lean against while you're working with weights. Doing weight workouts on a ball may feel a bit clumsy at first. But the work your body does to maintain your balance actually helps you to challenge your muscles more effectively. Exercising on the ball is especially good for the muscles in your core, such as your abdominals and back muscles. Read the box or label so that you're sure to choose a ball that is the right size for your height: Most women will require a ball that's fifty-five or sixty-five centimeters in diameter. Most are sold with easy-to-use pumps and take only a few minutes to inflate. If you haven't used a ball before, underinflate it slightly at first. If it's a bit soft, it will be easier to keep your balance. As you grow more accustomed to the ball, you can add more air to give yourself more of a challenge.

The ball is not absolutely necessary—most of the exercises designed for the ball can be performed standing, sitting in a chair, or lying on a mat.

My experience is that clients love the ball and can tell it produces results. It's suitable for any age and fitness level. It adds some fun to your strength workouts.

Before you begin the program, you'll want to keep a few key points in mind:

- *Always warm up* before you start lifting weights. Spend a few minutes getting your body temperature up and your blood flowing. This will help you prevent injury.

- *Lift and lower your weights slowly.* Make your muscles do the work. Don't use momentum and don't swing the weights around. If you can't lift a weight without swinging it, it's too heavy.

- *Breathe.* Don't hold your breath. Exhale during the hardest part of the exercise.

- *Don't stop halfway.* Make sure you're using full range of motion throughout the movement.

- *Keep your lower abdominal muscles tight to protect your back!* Pay attention to your posture and keep everything nice and tight to avoid injury.

WHICH COMES FIRST?

Clients often ask me which should come first—cardiovascular training or weights? My advice is to do whatever feels good and fits into your schedule. I tend to do my cardio first because it warms me up and gets me motivated. Others like to do their weights first so that they're not tired out from their cardio. In the fitness media, there are so many rules! But my opinion is—better to do it than not to do it at all.

I leave it up to you. You can even do it at different times of the day. There's no reason why you can't do your cardio in the morning and your weights at night. Remember, it's all cumulative!

GOING SLOW AND BEING PATIENT

One of the biggest mistakes beginners make is doing too much too soon. If you are new to weight training, your body isn't used to using your muscles in such an intense way. If you try to do too much too soon, you'll know it—your muscles will tell you all about it! Many a beginner has spent a miserable week trying to gingerly walk up the stairs because her legs were so sore. To avoid burning out, you need to prepare your body for building muscle by starting gradually. You should concentrate on learning proper technique and form, which exercises to do, which muscle groups to work, and how much weight to use.

Your body will also undergo other adjustments, gradually replacing lost body fat with muscle. You probably won't see drastic changes on the scale in the beginning. You might even gain a pound or two. But don't panic: You are rearranging your body composition, tightening and toning. If you don't like what you're seeing on the scale, don't give up. Simply use a better measuring stick, such as a measuring tape or a favorite pair of pants that has been too tight for the last three years!

HOW OFTEN SHOULD YOU LIFT WEIGHTS?

You may have heard that you shouldn't lift weights on consecutive days. But this advice applies primarily to weight lifters who are trying to make radical changes in their muscle mass. For less dramatic sculpting and toning, there really is nothing wrong with lifting weights every day as long as the muscle group you are working isn't sore. So if you are short on time and it works better for your schedule to do two days' worth of strength-training workouts over four days, go right ahead. You can do the upper body exercises on Monday and the lower body on Tuesday. Just don't work the same muscle group two days in a row if you feel any soreness.

Here's a very crude description of what weight training does: Lifting weights actually tears small fibers in your muscles. In the next twenty-four to forty-eight hours following a weight workout, those muscle fibers repair themselves, assuming that you've been eating enough protein and there are plenty of good nutrients available in your system. As those fibers get repaired, the muscle grows or plumps slightly. Over time, that effect is responsible for the sculpted look of well-toned muscle.

If your muscles are sore, that means you worked them hard and they need to repair before you go at it again. If they aren't sore at all, consider increasing the weight or adding another set to make a greater impact on your muscles. Everyone is different: A weight that challenges your exercise buddy might not have a noticeable impact on you.

As is the case with cardio, when your schedule is really crazy, remember that a little weightlifting is better than nothing at all. If you can't fit the entire strength-training routine into a particularly busy week, just pick two exercises per day. By the end of the week, you will have worked your whole body—maybe even twice—and you'll be doing those muscles and bones a favor.

BYE-BYE BULK

Please don't worry about building bulky muscles! This weight-training regimen will help you look smaller, not bigger. Remember, a pound of muscle takes up less space and has more density than a pound of fat. Whether or not your muscles become bigger (hypertrophy) depends on three factors: genetics, gender, and training intensity.

- The genetic influence on muscle size is mostly a matter of the type of muscle fibers you have. In other words, you're built pretty much like everyone else in your family.

- In terms of gender, men have greater amounts of testosterone and other hormones that influence muscle size with strength training. Women lack the hormones and bone structure required for the classic masculine bodybuilder physique.

- Training intensity is the factor you control! If you want bigger muscles, use heavier weights and do fewer repetitions, as few as eight per set. If you want to tone and tighten, use lighter weights and more repetitions.

THE MOTIVATING BODIES
MOVE TO LOSE STRENGTH PROGRAM

Week 1

- Start with one full-body workout for the week. You can either do one twenty-minute workout or split it into two ten-minute workouts. Select one ten-minute upper body routine and one ten-minute lower body routine from the following workouts to condition your entire body. These workouts have been designed to use each muscle group.

- If your week is so crazy, you can't fit in either a twenty-minute workout or two ten-minute workouts, try to do at least two exercises each day. Work a different muscle group each time. You could do your biceps and triceps on Monday, your shoulders on Tuesday, your chest on Wednesday, and divide the leg exercises between Thursday and Friday.

- Perform one set of 12 to 15 repetitions ("reps") of each exercise using weights that are appropriate for your strength level. By the last rep, your muscle should be fatigued. If the muscle isn't tired, increase the weight. If you can't complete 12 repetitions, use a lighter weight. As you get stronger, you may need to increase the weight to reach fatigue. To lose body fat and build muscle, you need to use enough weight so that you can only complete 12 to 15 repetitions for one to three sets. (Beginners should complete one set. Intermediate and advanced exercisers should complete two or three sets.) Rest for about thirty seconds between sets.

- You may be a little sore the next day or two. If so, rest for one or two days before strength training those same muscles again.

- Try to perform the full strength-training workout one time this week. Do two workouts this week if you want extra credit.

Week 2

- Continue the twenty-minute workouts as in Week 1, but add a second workout so that you're doing two per week, or the equivalent in mini-workouts. You can do two days of twenty minutes or four days of ten minutes or do two or three exercises every day.

- Perform one or two sets of 12 to 15 reps of each exercise using the appropriate weight. Add more weight (two to three pounds) when you can complete 15 reps without getting tired. If you have the time, you can also add additional sets.

Top 10 Quick One-Minute Moves to Add Muscle During the Day

1. *Squeeze and squat:* Do squats in the kitchen, while brushing your teeth, or while making the bed. Squats develop strength in your quads and glutes and burn calories all at once! See my Lower Body Workout #1 for tips on maintaining good form.

2. *Shop and curl:* As you shop, do some bicep curls. Lift your packages, handbag, or grocery basket several times in each arm while you make your purchase decisions!

3. *The stair climber:* A flight of stairs is like a stair stepper, at your disposal to tone your buns and legs! A 135-pound woman burns approximately ten calories per minute walking up an average flight of stairs. Increase your speed and you'll burn more. Use the stairs whenever possible.

4. *Doggie does it:* Take ten minutes to play with your pooch and tone your buns! Get down on all fours and lift your leg up behind you. Remember to squeeze the glutes as you lower and lift.

5. *Baby weights:* Let your baby help you strengthen your chest. Lie on your back, holding baby on your chest. Carefully lift her up to do your chest press and lower her back down. She'll enjoy it more than you.

6. *Do walking lunges during commercials:* The commercial breaks during an hour on nighttime TV total approximately fifteen minutes. Take a lap around the family room and work those legs during each break! See my Lower Body Workout #2 for tips on maintaining good form.

7. *Play ball:* Engage one of your kids or your spouse in a game of ball. Use a basketball or soccer ball and do some chest passes, overhead passes, and soccer kicks. You can even use the ball to make ab crunches more challenging. Have your partner toss you the ball as you curl up, and pass it back as you curl down in your crunch.

8. *Desk chair crunches:* Take a break each day to work those abs for one minute. Hold on to the sides of your chair, sit tall, engage those lower abs, and exhale as you lift your knees toward your chest. Hold for a moment, then lower.

9. *Push-ups:* This is a move you can take with you wherever you go! Get down on the floor or use the wall. Do a quick 10 every morning and 10 more every night! See my Upper Body Workout #1 for tips on maintaining proper form.

10. *Calf raises:* Holding on to a banister for balance, stand on one foot with the ball of your foot on the edge of a step. Press your heel downward, then lift yourself upward. Repeat several times for each leg.

Week 3

Continue with the work you've been doing from Week 2 but add a third day if you can fit it into your schedule. Add more weight (two to three pounds) if your muscles aren't feeling tired after a full set. Continue with the upper and lower body workouts to condition your entire body.

Week 4

In Week 4, add another set to your exercises. This will take a little extra time, perhaps an additional five minutes. If this is a problem, divide it up by doing a little each day. Schedule at least one day of rest between workouts if your muscles are sore.

WORKOUTS

Lower Body Workout #1:

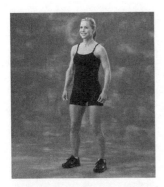

8.1 • Standing ready

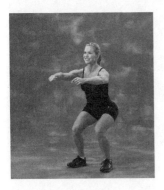

8.2 • Finished position

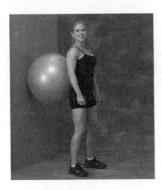

8.3 • Ball against the wall, starting position

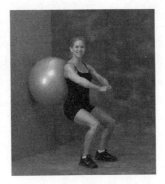

8.4 • Ball against the wall, finished position

The Basic Squat

(quads, hamstrings, glutes)

Stand with feet hip-width apart, abs tight (see figure 8.1). Bend your knees and lower your body into a squat position as low as you can go, but stop when your knees are at 90 degrees. Pretend you are sitting back into a chair—stick your buttocks out, keep your chest lifted and spine long—and keep your knees above your ankles (see figure 8.2). Push through the heels and squeeze your buttocks to lift back to starting position. For a more advanced exercise, hold a dumbbell in each hand. To protect your lower back, use your ball against a wall (see figure 8.3) and press into the ball, stabilizing your back (see figure 8.4). Repeat for a total of 15 squats.

Step-ups

(works the entire leg, including inner and outer thigh quads and glutes)

Using an athletic step or a kitchen step stool, place your right foot up on the step, making sure the whole foot, including the heel, is firmly placed (see figure 8.5). Using your right glute (*gluteus maximus,* the large muscle in your buttock), pull your body up onto the step so that you're standing on your right foot (see figure 8.6). Then slowly lower yourself back down, maintaining control. (Don't just let momentum drop your body.) Perform 15 repetitions with each leg. When this becomes easy, hold hand weights for an extra challenge. Pay attention to good posture and tighten your abs to protect your back.

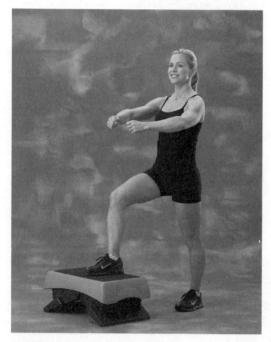

8.5 • Starting position

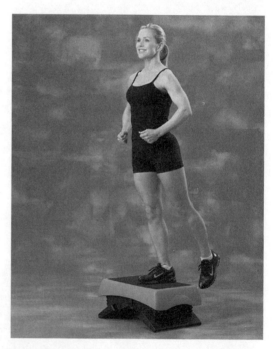

8.6 • Lifting onto the step

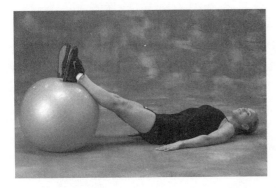

8.7 • Starting position

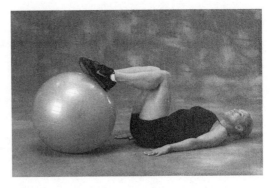

8.8 • Rolling the ball in toward the glutes

Hamstring Roll-ins with Ball

(one of my favorites)

Lie on your back and straighten your legs, with your heels resting on the ball (see figure 8.7). Press your heels into the ball as you contract your abs, bend your knees, and roll the ball in toward the glutes (see figure 8.8). Then roll back out to the starting position. To increase the difficulty, try lifting your hips off the floor and keeping them up the whole time (see figure 8.9), using the stabilizing muscles of your core to intensify the hamstring curl (see figure 8.10). Repeat 12 to 15 times.

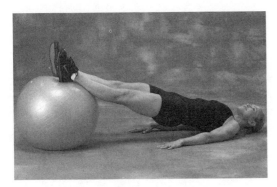

8.9 • Performing the exercise with lifted hips

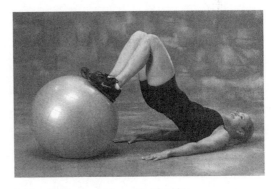

8.10 • Finished position with lifted hips

Bun Lift

(awesome for toning those buns)

Get down on all fours. Place a light weight behind your right knee and bend your leg to hold it in place. Flex your foot. Tighten your abs and flatten your back (see figure 8.11). Squeeze your butt muscles to lift your right leg until it is level with your hips (see figure 8.12). Lower. Repeat 12 to 15 times before switching sides.

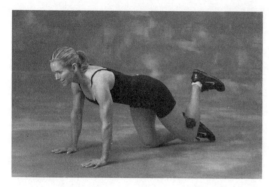

8.11 • Starting position

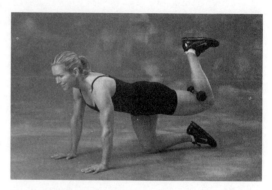

8.12 • Lifting the leg

Lower Body Workout #2

The Lunge

(another favorite; works the entire leg, including inner and outer thigh and calves)

Stand in split stance: right leg in front, right foot flat, left leg in back, heel off the ground (see figure 8.13). Bend both knees and lower into a lunge, keeping your front knee directly above the ankle and the back knee pointing down at the floor. Keep your abs tight, chest lifted, and spine long. Only lower your body as far as is comfortable. Don't bend your knees more than 90 degrees (see figure 8.14). Squeeze through your buns to raise yourself back up. For a more advanced exercise, hold dumbbells in your hands. Do 12 to 15 repetitions, then switch legs.

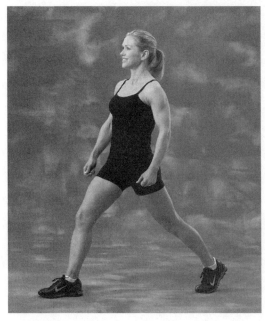

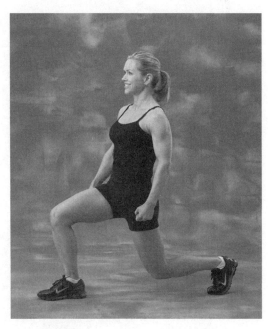

8.13 • Starting position

8.14 • Lowering the body

Side-lying Leg Lifts

(with ball)

Lie on your side with your torso on the ball. Your bottom leg is bent on the mat and your top leg is extended with the foot resting on the floor. Rest your top hand on your hip, and put your other arm over the ball, placing your hand on the floor for balance (see figure 8.15). Keeping abdominals tight to balance and stabilize your pelvis, lift your top leg as high as comfortably possible (see figure 8.16). Hold for a moment and then slowly lower. Keep your body in one plane with your abs tight—don't let the top hip rotate forward or back. (Imagine that your body is flattened against a sheet of glass.) Do 12 to 15 repetitions on each side.

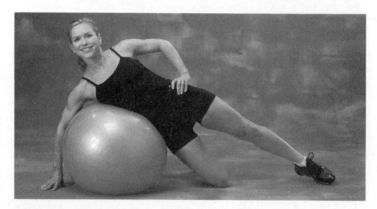

8.15 • Starting position

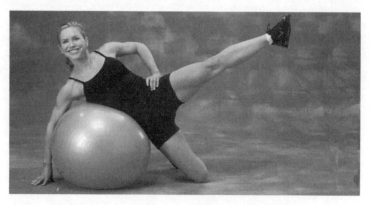

8.16 • Lifting the leg

Inner Thigh Squeezes

Sit on the floor, arms behind you, hands flat on the floor for support. With legs bent, place the ball between your knees, heels touching the ground. Keeping your abs contracted, squeeze the ball using your inner thighs (see figure 8.17). Do 10 slow squeezes followed by 10 quick squeezes. Relax and repeat several times.

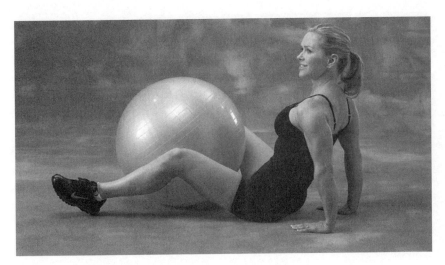

8.17 • Inner Thigh Squeeze

Prone Hip Extensions

Lie facedown on the ball with your abs on the ball. Place your hands on the floor in a push-up position. Keep your legs hip-width apart with your toes lightly touching the ground (see figure 8.18). With your abs contracted to support your lower back, contract the glutes and lift straight legs up in unison until they are in line with the rest of your body (see figure 8.19). Bend from your hips to return to starting position. If this is too challenging, start by lifting one leg at a time. Do 12 to 15 repetitions.

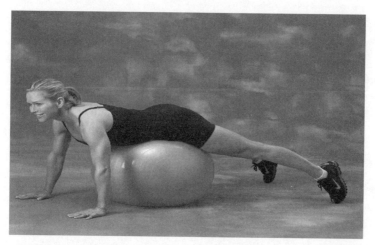

8.18 • Starting position

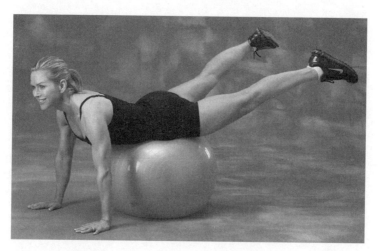

8.19 • Lifting the legs

Upper Body Workout #1:

Chest Press on Ball

Sit on the ball holding your hand weights. Roll your body forward to create a "weight bench." Keep your knees bent at 90 degrees, your thighs and torso parallel to the floor, and your feet shoulder-width apart. Contract your abs and glutes to support your torso. Your head, neck, and shoulders should rest comfortably on the ball. Bend your elbows at 90 degrees so that your arms are in the shape of a goalpost. Hold the weights above your chest, slightly toward your shoulders (see figure 8.20). Keeping your abs tight to protect the lower back, exhale and push your arms up overhead—keeping the weights a few inches apart. Don't lock your elbows (see figure 8.21). Lower and repeat. Do 12 to 15 reps.

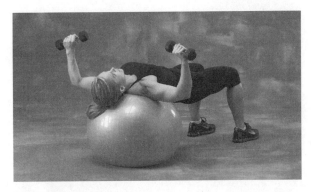

8.20 • Starting position

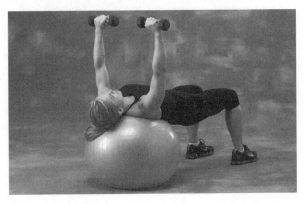

8.21 • Lifting the weights

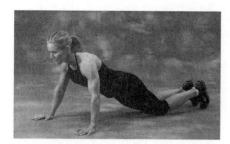

8.22 • Starting position, on knees

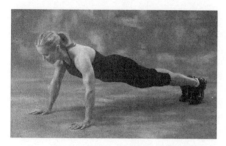

8.23 • Starting position, on toes

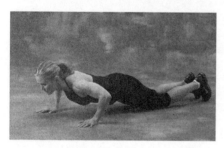

8.24 • Lowering the body from the knees

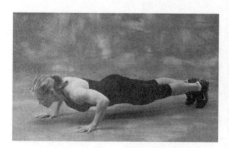

8.25 • Lowering the body from the toes

Push-ups

(chest, triceps, biceps)

Stretch out on the mat, facedown, with your arms straight in front of you and hands flat on the floor. Keep your hands under your shoulders and a little wider than shoulder-width apart. If you are a beginner, start on your knees (see figure 8.22). If you are more advanced, rest on your toes, keeping your core tight and level (see figure 8.23). Bend your elbows to a 90-degree angle and lower your body, keeping your abs tight. Don't sag in the middle (see figures 8.24 and 8.25). Push back to start and repeat 12 to 15 times.

A great modification for beginners is the *Wall Push-up:* Stand at arm's length from a wall. Place the palms of your hands on the wall in front of you at shoulder height, a few inches wider than your shoulders (see figure 8.26). Keeping your abs tight and back straight, bend your elbows and lower your body toward the wall until your elbows are at 90-degree angles (see figure 8.27). Return to start.

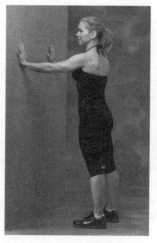

8.26 • Starting position against the wall

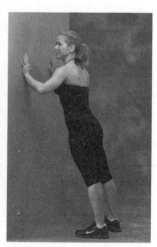

8.27 • Lowering the body against the wall

Triceps Overhead Press

Sit tall on the ball or stand with your feet hip-width apart. Clasp one dumbbell with both hands. Extend both arms straight overhead, with your elbows close to your ears (see figure 8.28). Bend your elbows and slowly lower the weight behind you. Keep your elbows in close to your ears (see figure 8.29). Contract your triceps (the muscles at the back of your upper arms) and straighten your elbows to return to start. Do 12 to 15 reps.

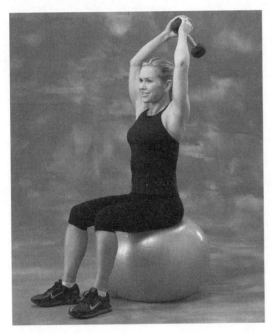

8.28 • Starting position

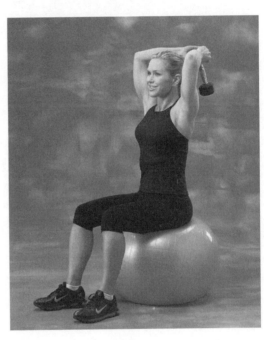

8.29 • Lowering the weight

Bicep Curls

Sit tall on the ball or stand with your feet hip-width apart, holding a dumbbell in each hand, palms facing out (see figure 8.30). Bend your elbows and slowly bring the weights toward your shoulders, keeping the elbows in tight to the body. Don't swing the weights (see figure 8.31). Lower the weights slowly and repeat. Keep your abs tight throughout the move. Do 12 to 15 reps.

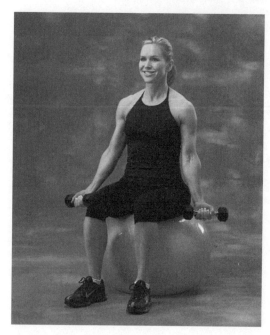

8.30 • Starting position

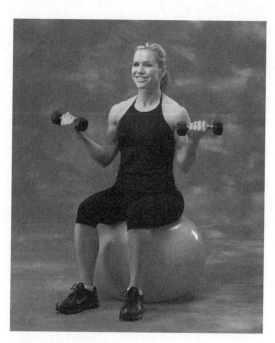

8.31 • Lifting the weights

Single Arm Row

(mid-back)

Hold a dumbbell in your left hand. Stand in split stance and place your right hand on the ball or the seat of a chair. Keep your torso and hips facing the floor, contracting the abs to protect and stabilize your lower back. Drop your left arm down straight to begin (see figure 8.32). Pull up the arm, bending your elbow and feeling the shoulder blade contract—imagine starting a lawn mower (see figure 8.33). Lower. Repeat 12 to 15 times per side.

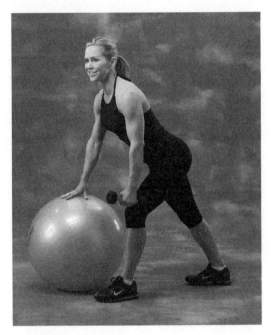

8.32 • Starting position

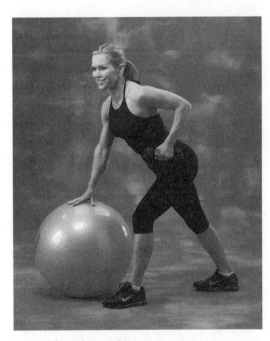

8.33 • Lifting the weight

Lateral Raise

(shoulders)

Stand with feet hip-width apart and hold the dumbbells at your sides, with your palms facing in (see figure 8.34). Keeping your elbows slightly bent, lift your arms straight up out to the sides, until they are parallel to the floor. Do not raise your arms above shoulder level (see figure 8.35). Lower your hands back to your sides. Keep your shoulders relaxed—don't shrug! If you are a beginner, do this exercise without any weight at first. Do 12 to 15 reps.

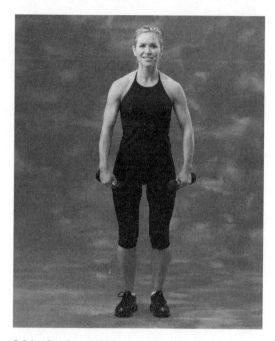

8.34 • Starting position

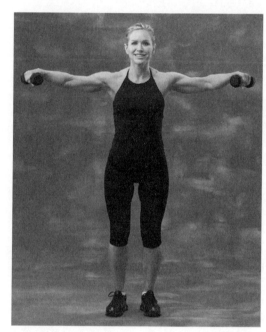

8.35 • Raising the arms

Upper Body Workout #2

Chest Flies on the Ball

Sit on the ball holding your hand weights. Roll your body forward to create a "weight bench." Keep your knees bent at a 90-degree angle, your thighs and torso parallel to the floor, and your feet shoulder-width apart. Contract your abs and glutes to support your torso. Your head, neck, and shoulders should rest comfortably on the ball. Begin with your arms straight up over your chest, palms facing each other (see figure 8.36). Slowly open your arms and lower them down to the sides. Go no lower than shoulder level and keep your elbows slightly bent at all times (see figure 8.37). Then lift your arms back to start. Imagine you are "hugging a tree trunk." Do 12 to 15 reps.

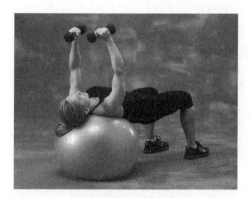

8.36 • Starting position

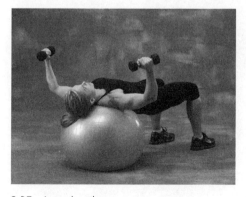

8.37 • Lowering the arms

Dumbbell Pullover

(back and chest)

Choose a moderate-weight dumbbell and lie face up on the ball. Roll your body forward to create a weight bench, holding the dumbbell straight up overhead at eye level. Keep your core stable (see figure 8.38). With a slow, controlled motion, lower the weight behind your head, keeping your arms slightly bent, going only as far back as is comfortable (see figure 8.39). Squeeze your back to pull the weight back up to start. Repeat 12 to 15 times.

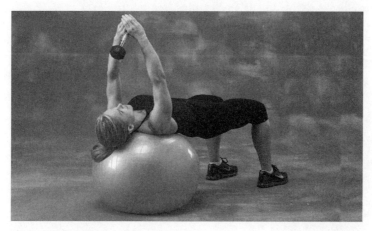

8.38 • Starting position

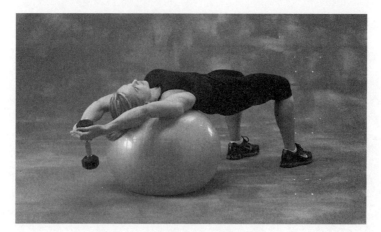

8.39 • Lowering the weight

Triceps Dips

Sit on a step, chair, or ball with your hands next to your thighs, fingertips pointing toward your knees. Lift your buttocks off the seat and move your body so that it's slightly in front of the seat or ball. Keep your knees slightly bent (see figure 8.40). Bend from the elbows and lower your body a few inches. This will feel a bit like sliding down a wall. Keep your shoulders relaxed and the elbows pointing back (see figure 8.41). Push back up to starting position and repeat 12 to 15 times.

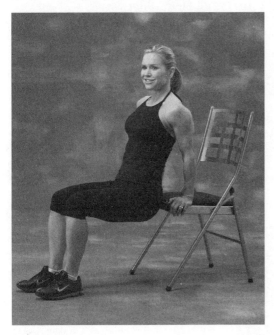

8.40 • Starting position

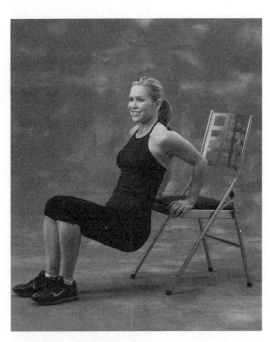

8.41 • Bending the elbows

Bicep Preacher Curls

With a weight in each hand, lean your torso into the ball, legs extended behind you, abs tight to protect your lower back (see figure 8.42). (If this position is too difficult, you can drop your knees to the floor for extra support—see figure 8.43.) Bring your arms forward over the ball, holding the hand weights with your palms facing up. Pressing your elbows into the ball, bend them and bring the weights toward the shoulders (see figure 8.44). Go slowly, maintaining control throughout the movement. Lower weights back to start to complete the full range of motion.

Repeat 12 to 15 times.

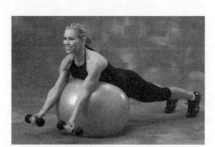

8.42 • Starting position

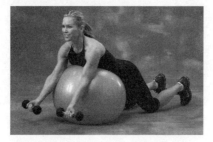

8.43 • Starting position, on knees

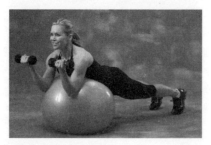

8.44 • Lifting the weights

Rear Delt

(back of the shoulders)

With a weight in each hand, lean your torso into the ball, legs extended behind you, abs tight to protect your lower back (see figure 8.45). (If this position is too difficult, you can drop your knees to the floor for extra support—see figure 8.46.) Drop your arms toward the floor. Squeeze your shoulder blades together as you lift the weights, extending your arms out to the sides like an airplane (see figure 8.47). Make sure to relax your neck. Don't squeeze or scrunch the shoulders. Return to start and repeat 12 to 15 times.

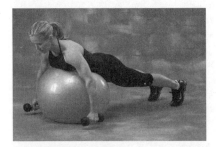

8.45 • Starting position

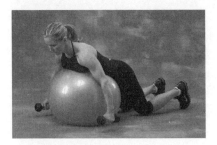

8.46 • Starting position, on knees

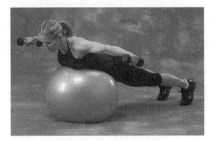

8.47 • Lifting the weights

Overhead Press

(shoulders)

Sit tall on the ball, or stand, holding hand weights in both hands. Begin with your arms bent in "goalpost" position, at 90-degree angles with straight wrists and tight abs (see figure 8.48). Lift your arms overhead until they are straight (see figure 8.49). Lower back to the goalpost position. Repeat 12 to 15 times.

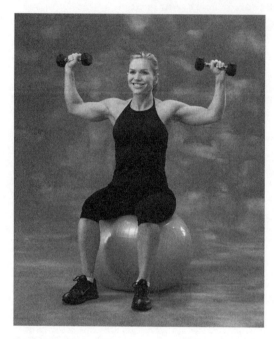

8.48 • Starting position

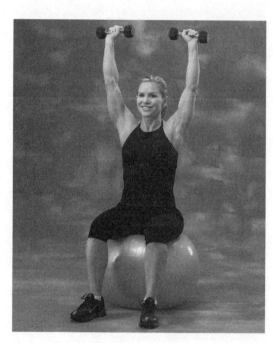

8.49 • Lifting the weights

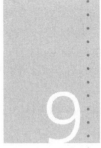

Core Capabilities: The Core-Strengthening Workout

9

If you don't concentrate, you'll end up on your rear.

—TAI BABILONIA

When it comes to physical activity, what is your style? Have you hated exercise most of your life? Do you go from one workout craze to the next? Maybe you are a weekend warrior—someone who does nothing physical all week and then acts like an Olympian on the weekend. Maybe you are fairly fit? No matter what your exercise personality or fitness level, Pilates will work for you:

- It can improve your posture.
- It builds long, lean muscle without bulk.
- It improves strength, coordination, balance, flexibility, and joint mobility.
- It firms and tightens the abdominal muscles that strengthen and protect the spine.

Pilates is a fitness discipline that values quality over quantity. It's a series of controlled, thoughtful, focused movements, each engineered to deliver results. The mindfulness you bring to your Pilates practice will be reflected in your ability to perform your everyday activities with greater ease. You will also notice—and appreciate—your flatter, tighter midsection and stronger spine!

The exercise ball brings new dimension and functionality to traditional Pilates exercises. As you make dozens of tiny adjustments—some deliberate, others unconscious—to keep your balance, your body engages and challenges all the muscles in your torso and back. The ball will help you engage a whole new set of stabilizing muscles, making weak muscles strong and strong muscles more stable. Adding the ball enhances the Pilates experience. The ball will help you be more aware of your body in space and enhance your sense of balance.

With or without the ball, Pilates is as much a mental regimen as a physical one. Like yoga, which we will discuss in the next chapter, Pilates is considered to be a true mind-body discipline. Concentration is critical to your success. Proper breathing is fundamental, helping you to relax and make the movements more effective. Unlike traditional calisthenics, Pilates is not just countless, mindless repetitions. There is a clear purpose and breathing pattern behind each exercise.

STRENGTH IN BALANCE

Many of us are starting to understand that the key to health is balance: Balance between inner and outer, moderate and extreme, doing and not doing. We need to find balance between what we can accomplish and what we cannot by finding balance and harmony in our bodies. Once we attain a sense of body balance, we can transfer that feeling to our relationships and life habits.

Balance is control. I always tell my clients and classes that exercise is the one thing we can control during the day. When everything else seems so out of control, exercise is our chance for accomplishment. Even if you are a perfectionist, you cannot control everything. The unexpected occurs—we slip on ice, we miss a step, and we have an accident. These kinds of things happen to anyone, no matter how careful, strong, or graceful. Then there are the emotional things we cannot control—like traffic, sick kids, bills, and deadlines. But better body balance makes it easier to cope, helps us to prevent injury, and provides a foundation for the emotional balance we need to pull us through the crises of our daily lives.

Balance is "use it or lose it" in principle. If you are sedentary, you will tend to lose your balance as you get older. Fortunately, it doesn't have to be a losing battle. You can improve your coordination and practice your balance with Pilates at any age. It will help you, literally, to stay on the ball!

MEET THE MUSCLES

What, exactly, is your core? It's your midsection, your front, back, and sides. These are the major muscles of your abdominals group (see figure 9.1):

- *Obliques:* The internal and external obliques are located on the side and front of the abdomen, around your waist. They are responsible for twisting motions and stability.

- *Rectus Abdominus:* The *rectus abdominus* is your "crunching" muscle, a long muscle that extends along the front of the abdomen. This muscle, when well developed, is the "six-pack" that becomes visible with reduced body fat.

- *Transverse Abdominus (TVA):* The deepest of the abdominal muscles, the TVA muscles act like a belt, wrapping around your spine for protection and stability. These are the muscles most of us complain about as we age because when they are weak and neglected, they are responsible for the dreaded "pouch problem." They are located just below the navel. To locate your TVA, lie down and make a coughing sound. Then inhale and on the exhale, pretend you're zipping up a pair of tight jeans as you scoop the abs in toward the spine. The muscle you contract is your *transverse abdominus.*

Your spine is also an important part of your core—including:

- Seven vertebrae in your neck (cervical spine)
- Twelve vertebrae in your midback (thoracic spine)
- Five vertebrae in your lower back (lumbar spine)

BACK PAIN BASICS

Back pain is common because so many muscles have to contract and relax to allow you to stand and move. Your spine was made to go front and back, side to side. The best way to keep it supple is to flex and extend the spine and the muscles that support it every day. Movement keeps all your vertebrae lubricated and well supplied with blood.

Maintaining good posture during everyday activities and proper alignment during exercise will go a long way toward alleviating the pressures that cause back pain. Exercise also helps you keep your back's supporting cast in good condition. Your tendons attach muscles to bones, ligaments hold your vertebrae together, and muscles protect your spine and hold your body in place. If all of these are healthy and strong, you're in business. But if you have weak muscles, poor posture, and/or excess weight, your back will be one of the first places you feel the strain.

If you suffer from back pain, don't start exercising until you visit your doctor to rule out major injuries. If your physician gives you the okay, you can get busy strengthening your torso. Exercise will help, of course. But your first step is posture.

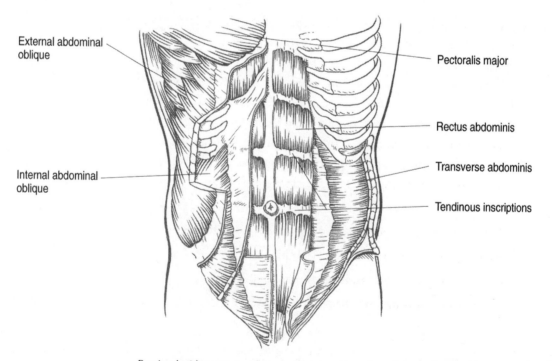

Reprinted with permission from the American Council on Exercise (2003). *ACE Personal Trainer Manual, 3rd Edition.* San Diego: American Council on Exercise. www.acefitness.org.

A POSTURE PRIMER

If you've ever worked with a trainer or used an exercise video, you've probably heard the phrase "proper form." This usually refers to your posture as you're doing an exercise. Even when you're not working out, proper form can protect you from injury all day long.

Good posture includes several vital elements:

- A fairly straight line from your ears, shoulders, hips, knees, and ankles
- Your head centered, front to back and side to side
- Even shoulders, hips, and knees, with neither side higher nor lower than the other

Some of the most common posture mistakes include:

- A head that sags forward
- Rounded shoulders
- Arched lower back
- Excessive anterior pelvic tilt (flat back)
- Excessive posterior pelvic tilt (sway back)

To figure out if you have good posture, take a good look at yourself in a full-length mirror. Check to see if:

- Your head is straight
- Your shoulders are level
- Your hips are level
- Your kneecaps face the front
- Your ankles are straight

Now look at yourself from the side (even better: have someone else evaluate you) and look for the following:

- Your head is straight rather than slumped forward or backward
- Your chin is parallel to the floor
- Your shoulders are in line with your ears

- Your knees are straight
- There is a slight forward curve to your lower back

Once you identify your posture imperfections, you can start working on them. But don't worry—nobody's perfect. Your first step is to be aware of your posture throughout the day, while standing, sitting at work, and driving in your car.

Beyond simple awareness, there are other corrective measures you can take. For example, if your head slumps forward and you have rounded shoulders, you probably have tight chest muscles and weak upper back muscles. We can correct that with stretching out the chest and strengthening the upper back muscles. If you have an excessive pelvic tilt, strengthening the *transverse abdominus* muscles will help.

THE MOTIVATING BODIES MOVE TO LOSE CORE PROGRAM

This Pilates-inspired core body workout is designed for the healthy, active exerciser. The key is to work at your level.

Pilates is a very time-efficient form of exercise. You can opt to do the full ten-minute workout that follows or simply pick two or three exercises to do daily. As you will see on the workout schedules in chapter 11, I've suggested two workouts a week. But if you fall in love with Pilates, as I have, do it every day.

Pilates training offers benefits to every exerciser. The beginner, working at his or her level, can use modifications. Even the overweight and the very sedentary can start by doing modified versions of these exercises on a floor mat, graduating to using the ball as their strength improves.

Modify these exercises to work with your body. Muscle fatigue—the "Wow, I'm really feeling it" sensation—is fine. It's actually the goal of this workout. But these exercises are not supposed to hurt. Never work through pain.

Always consult your doctor before beginning a new workout regimen. Think quality of movement not quantity of repetitions. It's perfectly fine to modify this routine to your body's abilities, stopping short of the full range of motion until your body adapts and strengthens.

Remember to begin each exercise by contracting the *transverse ab-*

dominus first. Never push your abs out but rather draw or scoop them in toward your spine. Pilates instructors are always reminding their students, "Belly to the spine."

And remember to breathe. It will help you relax and get deeper into your stretches and movements. Never hold your breath.

No shoes are required. All you need is some open space, an exercise ball, and a mat!

Warm-up Stretches

Shell Stretch

(breathing practice)

Kneel on all fours. Place your hands shoulder-width apart and your knees hip-width apart. Sit your hips back into the heels and extend your arms forward, reaching your fingertips as far as you can without scrunching your shoulders. Rest your forehead onto the floor. Relax the neck, face, and shoulders. Keep the arms stretched and the fingers reaching (see figure 9.1). Take 10 to 15 deep, slow breaths. Feel the rib cage expand through the sides and back as you inhale; draw the belly to the spine as you exhale.

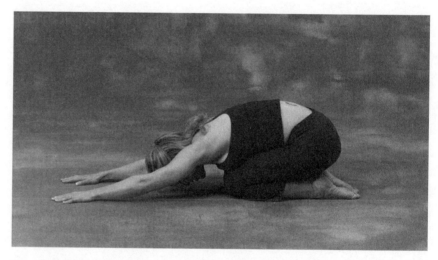

9.1 • Shell Stretch

Cat Stretch

(back flexion)

Kneel on all fours. Place your hands shoulder-width apart and your knees hip-width apart. Exhale and tuck your tailbone under, round the spine, and drop your head, as though you are looking for your navel (see figure 9.2). Push evenly through the hands and the knees and arch the upper back toward the sky (see figure 9.3). Hold for one complete breath and continue into Cow Stretch.

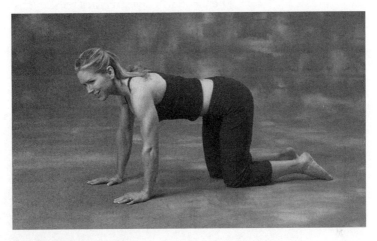

9.2 • Starting position

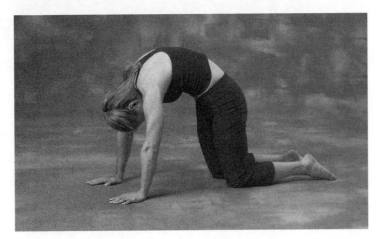

9.3 • Arching the back

Cow Stretch

(back extension)

Continue from Cat Sretch into back extension. Place your hands shoulder-width apart and your knees hip-width apart. Extend the spine, lift the tail-bone toward the sky, and drop the belly down toward the floor. Look up. Try to lengthen the crown of your head away from your tailbone (see figure 9.4). Hold for one complete breath and go back to the Cat Stretch. Repeat sequence 3 to 5 times.

Note: The Cat and Cow stretches release tension and increase mobility in the spine. Remember to hold your lower abs (*transverse abdominus*) in toward your spine.

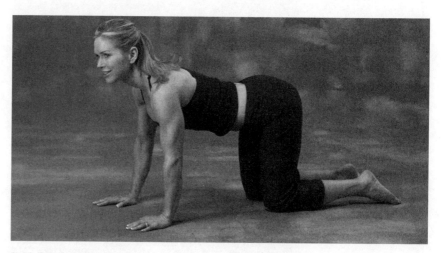

9.4 • Cow Stretch

Side Bend

(lateral flexion)

Kneel on the floor or sit tall on your ball with a neutral pelvis—tilting neither forward nor back. With arms extended straight overhead and shoulders relaxed away from the ears, inhale and reach up. Exhale as you bend your body to the right (see figure 9.5). To keep your torso in alignment, try imagining that you are flattened against a pane of glass. Feel the stretch up the entire side of the body. Visualize your spine hooking over like a candy cane. Inhale and straighten back to center. Exhale as you bend to the other side. Repeat 3 to 5 times on each side.

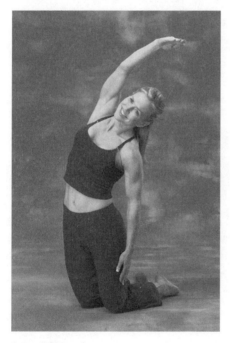

9.5 • Side Bend

Abs Stretch over Ball

Begin in a supine position with your head and shoulders on the exercise ball. Keep your knees directly over your ankles and your arms relaxed at your sides (see figure 9.6). Inhale slowly and stretch back on the ball, raising your arms gently over your head (see figure 9.7). Try to hold this position for 20 to 40 seconds. If you find this too difficult, just cut back on the number of seconds you hold the stretch and the range of motion.

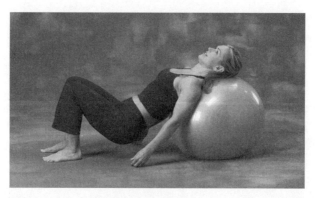

9.6 • Starting position

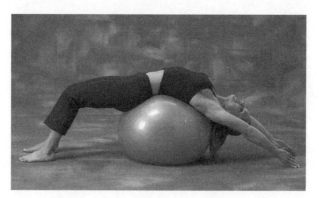

9.7 • The stretch

Exercises

Spinal Balance

Kneel on all fours. Place your hands shoulder-width apart and your knees hip-width apart. Keep your wrists under your shoulders and your knees under your hips. Draw your navel into your spine and stretch the crown of your head away from your tailbone. Keep your torso square to the ground (imagine balancing a cup of tea on your back—see figure 9.8). Exhale and extend your right arm and left leg, reaching your fingertips out and squeezing your glute muscle (see figure 9.9). Hold for two seconds and inhale as you lower. Repeat using your right arm and left leg. Continue alternating a total of 5 times on each side. (Remember to balance that cup of tea, keeping the back neutral and stable as you keep the navel pulled in toward your spine.)

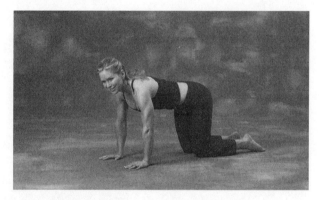

9.8 • Starting position

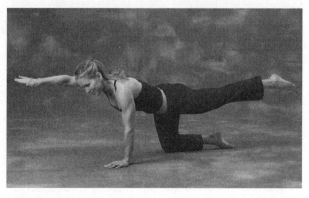

9.9 • The stretch

The Hundred on the Ball

Be sure to always initiate that navel-to-spine connection by engaging the transverse abdominus! Lie on your back with your arms by your sides. Rest your heels and calves on the exercise ball. (If this is too difficult, bend your knees to a 90-degree angle.) Sequentially lift first your head, then your shoulders off the mat. Gaze at your knees. Your head, neck, and shoulders stay relaxed (see figure 9.10). (If you are a beginner, you can modify this workout by putting your head down at any time during the exercise if you feel stress in the upper body.) Take five short, consecutive inhales, followed by five short, consecutive exhales. At the same time, lift your arms off the mat and pulse them, palms facing down, in unison with the breath. Repeat 10 times for a total of one hundred breaths.

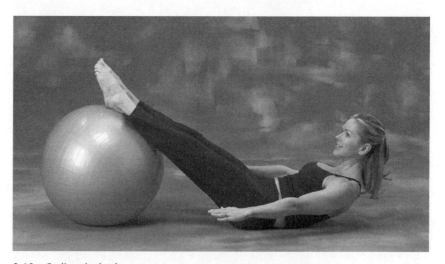

9.10 • Curling the body

Full Body Roll Up

Be sure to initiate the navel-to-spine connection, engaging the transverse abdominus! Lie on your back with your legs extended and your arms relaxed and stretched overhead (see figure 9.11). Engage those abdominal muscles as you inhale and stretch your arms up toward the sky (see figure 9.12). Exhale, lengthen the back of your neck, tuck your chin to your chest, pull the navel to the spine, and curl forward with your arms extending in front of you. Visualize leading with the top of your head in a "C" curve; curl forward until you are reaching for your toes (see figure 9.13). If you are just beginning, stop when your hands touch your knees. Inhale as you stay rounded. Begin reversing your direction, uncurling your body. Exhale as you continue to "drip" your spine back to the floor, one vertebra at a time, slowly lowering down. Repeat 5 to 8 times.

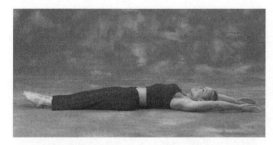

9.11 • Starting position

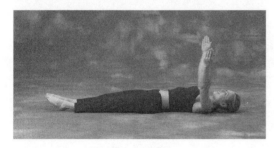

9.12 • Stretching the arms overhead

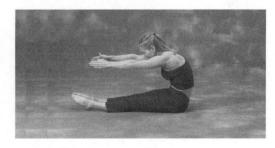

9.13 • Rolling up

Rolling Like a Ball

Be sure to initiate the navel-to-spine connection, engaging the transverse abdominus! Start seated on the floor, with your knees bent in toward your chest and hands relaxed onto calves. (Beginners can clasp their hands under their thighs and give them a hug.) Round your entire spine from the neck to the tailbone into a C-shaped curve and position yourself so that you're balancing just behind your sits bones (see figure 9.14). Inhale and roll back to your shoulder blades (see figure 9.15). Never roll onto your neck or head. Exhale to roll back up into a seated position, trying not to touch your feet to the floor. Intensely grip those low abs (navel to the spine) to maintain your "C" curve and balance. Imagine making an impression of each vertebra on the floor as you roll down. Repeat 8 to 10 times.

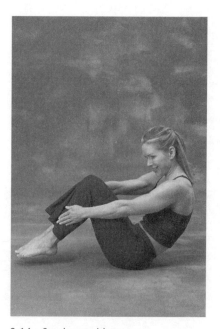

9.14 • Starting position

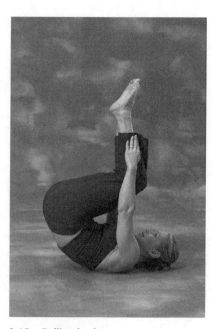

9.15 • Rolling back

Pilates Abdominal Crunch on the Ball

Be sure to initiate the navel-to-spine connection, engaging the transverse abdominus! Sit with the exercise ball under your hips, lower back, and middle back. (Roll the ball to the position that feels most comfortable for your level. The more your spine is in contact with the ball, the easier it will feel.) The wider the distance between your feet, the easier it will be to balance. Rest your hands on your thighs (see figure 9.16). Visualize sliding your rib cage to your pelvis as you lift your mid-back off the ball. Remember to sequentially roll up, lengthening through the back of the neck, chin slightly to the chest, and pull the navel to the spine. Your low back and hips remain touching the ball (see figure 9.17). Release and repeat 8 to 10 times. *Variation:* To engage your oblique muscles, add a slight twist to the torso.

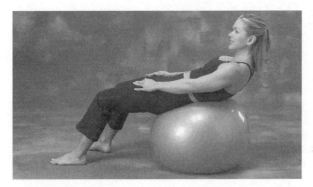

9.16 • Starting position

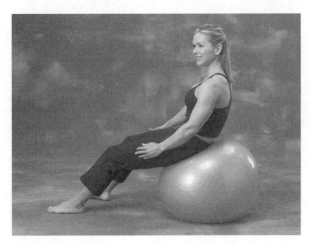

9.17 • The crunch

Double Leg Stretch with Ball

Be sure to initiate the navel-to-spine connection, engaging the transverse abdominus! Lie on your back on the floor with your knees bent at a 90-degree angle, soles of your feet on the ball (see figure 9.18). Sequentially lift your head and shoulders off the mat with your hands at your sides. (Modify by putting your head down at any time throughout the exercise if you feel stress in the upper body.) Inhale and stretch your body long, extending your arms overhead and pushing the ball out to lengthen the legs (see figure 9.19). Exhale and swim your arms back around to your sides and draw the knees back in a 90-degree angle (see figure 9.20). Inhale to stretch and exhale to draw in. Repeat this 5 to 10 times.

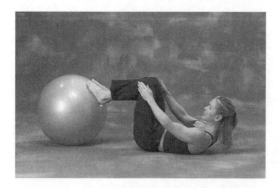

9.18 • Starting position

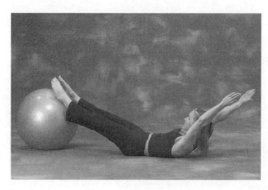

9.19 • The stretch

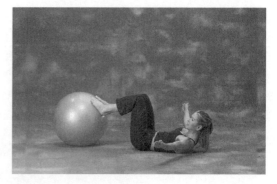

9.20 • Swimming the arms back to the sides

Spine Stretch Forward Seated on the Ball

(or on the floor)

Sit tall on your ball (or the floor) with a neutral pelvis—tilted neither forward nor back. Place your feet shoulder-width apart and keep your arms relaxed at your sides (see figure 9.21). Inhale, tightening your abs and extending your arms out in front of you as you peel your spine off an imaginary wall and stretch toward your toes (see figure 9.22). Start with your head rolling down one vertebra at a time to create a "C" curve. Inhale as you roll back up, stacking each vertebra back against that imaginary wall. Start at the lower back and stack your spine up like dominoes. Your shoulders, neck, and head should come up last. Repeat 5 to 8 times.

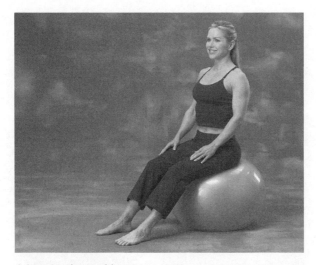

9.21 • Starting position

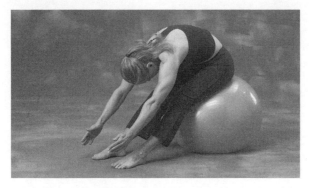

9.22 • The Spine Stretch

Spine Twist Seated on the Ball

(or the floor)

Sit tall on your ball with a neutral pelvis—tilted neither forward nor backward. Extend your arms out in front of you at shoulder height (see figure 9.23). Inhale, tightening your abs, lifting your chest, and sliding your shoulders slightly back. Exhale as you turn your torso to the left side. To engage your obliques, twist from your waist, not your hips. Visualize twisting the cap off a water bottle. Keep your head in alignment with your shoulders and upper body and your eyes focused on your left hand as it twists back (see figure 9.24). Inhale to return to center. Exhale and repeat on the right side. Continue alternating twists, 5 to 8 on each side.

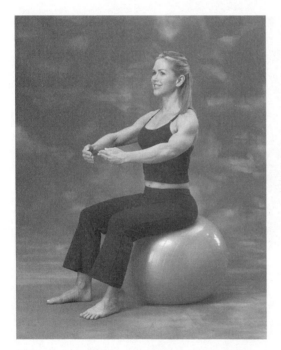

9.23 • Starting position

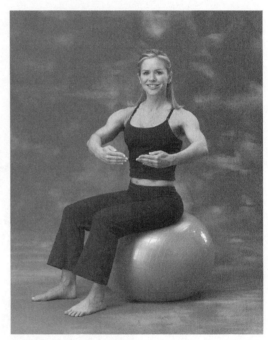

9.24 • The Spine Twist

Shoulder Bridge on Ball

Lie on the floor on your back with the soles of your feet on the exercise ball and your legs bent at a 90-degree angle. Keep your arms at your sides, palms down, and your shoulders relaxed (see figure 9.25). Inhale and lift your hips in the air like a drawbridge (see figure 9.26). Keep your hips steady facing the sky, and your navel pulled in to the spine, activating your *transverse abdominus* to protect your lower back. Exhale as you lower your back to the floor, as steady and stable as you can be. You can use your hands for balance, but try not to use them to push yourself up. Do not arch the spine; keep your abs scooped in toward the spine throughout. Beginners should try this without the ball, feet on the floor. Repeat 5 to 8 times.

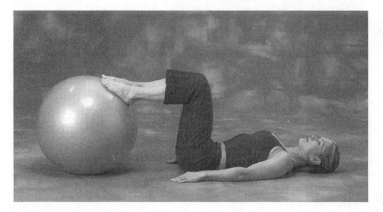

9.25 • Starting position

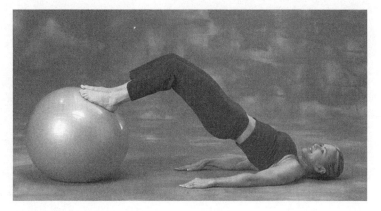

9.26 • Lifting the hips

Swan on Ball

Lie facedown with your pelvis and rib cage on the exercise ball and your fingers and toes touching the floor (see figure 9.27). Inhale to begin. Exhale as you draw your navel to the spine and raise your arms in front of you, lifting your chest off the ball. Inhale and imagine extending your spine, extending your head toward the sky, and sliding your tailbone down toward your heels (see figure 9.28). Exhale as you return to the starting position. Think of lengthening the spine rather than overarching it. Beginners should keep their hands on the ball and place their feet against a wall for stability (see figure 9.29). Repeat 5 to 8 times.

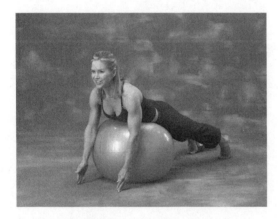

9.27 • Starting position

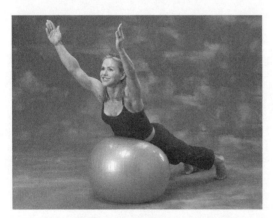

9.28 • The extension

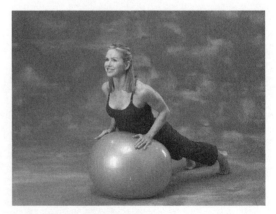

9.29 • The extension, with hands on the ball

Flex Time:
Yoga and Other Stretches

10

*When we are unable to find tranquility with-
in ourselves, it is useless to seek it elsewhere.*
—FRANÇOIS DE LA ROCHEFOUCAULD

When I first encountered yoga, I thought it was an interesting way to stretch. Today, I consider yoga to be one of my essentials for mental, as well as physical, well-being.

As I aged through my thirties, I started realizing that I just couldn't ignore my muscles after a long run. If I didn't take time to stretch, I would pay for it the next day, sometimes even a few hours later. My hips and hamstrings would get so tight, I felt as though I couldn't even stand up straight. But I didn't really take stretching seriously until a very painful hamstring injury gave me a wake-up call I couldn't ignore. I realized that my ligaments, tendons, and muscles were all getting older, and I needed to take care of them. So I started looking into yoga.

People who know me even a little bit recognize me as a classic type A, high-energy personality. So my friends and acquaintances couldn't believe that I, who could barely sit still for five minutes, would be able to get through an entire yoga class. But after a couple of classes, something miraculous began to happen. I realized how much my body, mind, and spirit were craving the relaxation, the peacefulness, and the ability to self-reflect. As busy as we all are, entire days, even weeks, can go by without any time for relaxation. I always ask the people in my classes: If you weren't taking yoga, would you take any time for yourself, for reflection, today?

What keeps me doing yoga now is the personal therapy it gives me. Yoga teaches us to be patient in stressful situations. Yoga promotes balanced thinking. It's often been said, "If you want to know how your yoga practice is going, take a look at your personal relationships." I truly believe that yoga makes me a better parent, spouse, friend, and person!

THE LATEST FIVE-THOUSAND-YEAR-OLD FITNESS FAD

Yoga—as a practice for the body, mind, and spirit—dates back five thousand years. Yet it's perfect for the way we live today. In the twenty-first century, yoga has entered the fitness mainstream and all kinds of everyday people are giving it a try. Yoga can be gentle or challenging, strictly physical or profoundly spiritual. It all depends on what you bring to your yoga practice and what you want to get from it. Here are just a few reasons why yoga is becoming so popular:

- It improves mood.
- It promotes relaxation.
- It increases range of motion.
- It can reduce pain in joints.
- It strengthens bones.
- It improves blood circulation.
- It promotes clearer thinking and deep concentration.
- It enhances self-awareness.
- It increases confidence as you master new poses.
- It rejuvenates the spine and central nervous system.
- It improves balance.
- It massages glands and organs.

MIND, BODY, AND BREATH

Yoga's combination of stretching and relaxing benefits makes it well worth your time. As we age, we need to lengthen, lubricate, and stretch our muscles after cardio exercise to reduce the chance of injury. And as we take on more and more responsibilities and stresses, the immediate benefits of even short periods of relaxation are obvious. A few moments snatched away from the cares and pressures of the world will leave you better equipped to tackle even the toughest to-do list.

Yoga allows both body and mind to rejuvenate, readying you for whatever challenges the day may bring. This is why I love to start my day with yoga. It prepares me to have a more balanced and even-tempered day. But yoga is just as beneficial in the evening, helping you to unwind, release tension, and sleep more peacefully.

At any time of day, yoga helps you relieve even the stresses you don't know you have! Often, when we aren't consciously aware of stress, our muscles will contract involuntarily. After you spend a long day sitting in traffic, sitting at your desk, and sitting in front of the television, the combination of slumped posture, tense shoulders, and lack of activity can really take its toll on your body.

Symptoms of stress also show up in your breathing. Anxiety tends to cause shallow breathing, which reduces the brain's oxygen supply and, unfortunately, exacerbates the anxiety. That's why common sense tells us to take a deep breath when we're tense. Deep, slow breathing can truly create a calming, cleansing, and nourishing effect for both body and mind.

Being mindful of the breath is a fundamental aspect of yoga. The practice known as Pranayama breathing consists of breathing in and out through your nose, creating a vacuumlike space in the back of the throat. Instead of sucking the air through the nostrils, you open up your airways and breathe. This technique is often called whisper breathing because of the noise it makes.

If you are trying to lose weight, breathing is an often overlooked ally. After all, weight loss is a matter of increasing metabolism and making it more efficient. Metabolism requires oxygen. So proper breathing can help.

Like all forms of exercise, the benefits of yoga are cumulative. The more you practice, the better you feel.

Yoga poses are called asanas. The gentle, low-impact postures in the following workout will help you stretch and tone your muscles, lubricate your joints, and keep your ligaments and tendons healthy.

THE MOTIVATING BODIES MOVE TO LOSE FLEXIBILITY PROGRAM

In the exercise programs outlined in chapter 11, I recommend doing yoga at least once a week for survival, two times a week for sanity, and three times a week for serenity.

Asanas—Working Poses

Warrior 1

Step forward with your right foot, bending your right knee and keeping your hips squared, facing in the same direction as your bent knee. Keep your left leg straight, foot flat, and toes slightly angled. Keep your feet about three or four feet apart (see figure 10.1). Exhale and deepen the lunge, with your heels aligned and abs tight. Keep the bent knee over the ankle. Sweep your arms overhead and look up, extending your spine (see figure 10.2). Hold for 4 to 6 breaths and repeat on the other side.

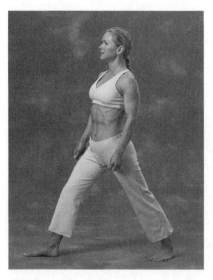

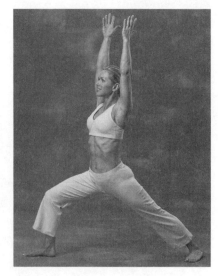

10.1 • Starting position

10.2 • Warrior 1

Warrior 2

Step forward with your right foot, bending your right knee and turning your hips to the side. Keep your head turned to the side (see figure 10.3). Stretch your arms straight out, keeping them parallel to the floor, with your shoulder blades relaxed and palms down. Keep your left leg straight, foot flat, toes slightly angled. Your feet should be around three to four feet apart (see figure 10.4). Exhale and deepen the lunge, with your heels aligned and your abs tight. Keep the bent knee over the ankle, with your torso upright and your spine long. Hold for 4 to 6 breaths and repeat on the other side.

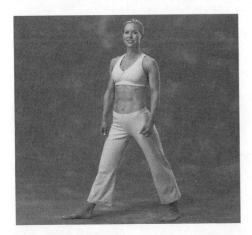

10.3 • Starting position

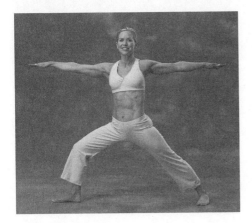

10.4 • Warrior 2

Tree Pose

This is a balancing pose. Stand with your feet hip-width apart, spine aligned, hands in prayer position (see figure 10.5). Shift your weight over to the left side and slowly lift the right leg and place the sole of the foot on the inside of the opposite ankle, knee, or inner thigh. Press the right knee back while keeping your hips steady. Find an object in front of you to focus on. Get your balance and hold, then push arms overhead, like the limbs of a tree, shoulders relaxed away from your ears (see figure 10.6). Hold this pose for four to six breaths and repeat on the other side.

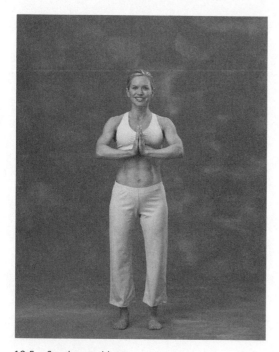

10.5 • Starting position

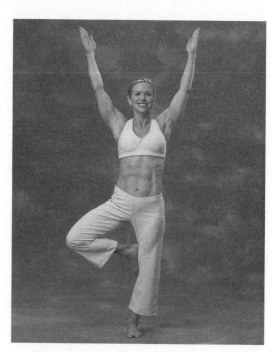

10.6 • Tree pose

Chair Pose

Standing with your feet hip-width apart, arms at your sides, bend both knees and sit back, sinking into your heels as if you were sitting into a chair. Engage the quads, glutes, and core body to balance. Sweep your arms overhead, next to your ears, and keep your chest and torso lifted and long (see figure 10.7). Hold for 4 to 6 breaths.

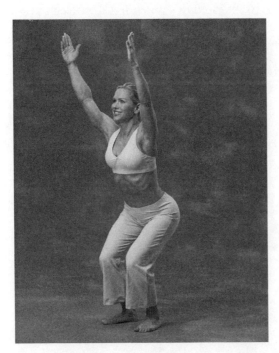

10.7 • Chair pose

Downward Facing Dog

Begin on your hands and knees. Place your feet hip-width apart, with your toes tucked under. Place your hands on the floor shoulder-width apart and spread your fingers (see figure 10.8). Straighten your legs and lift your tailbone toward the sky while pulling your navel toward the spine and gently pushing down through the heels (feel the stretch through the back of the legs). Open the upper back by rotating the shoulder blades slightly out. Keep the shoulders away from the ears and relax your head between your ears (see figure 10.9). Hold this pose for 4 to 6 deep breaths.

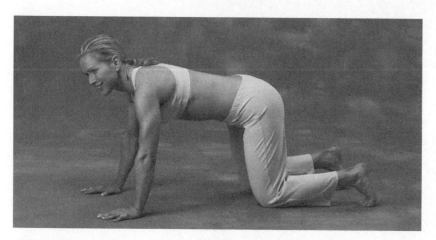

10.8 • Starting position

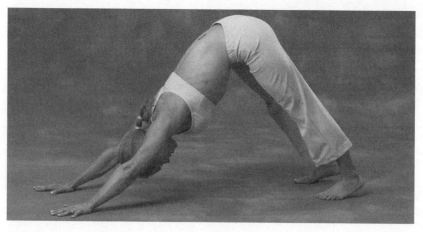

10.9 • Downward Facing Dog

Cobra

Lie facedown on the floor. Place your feet hip-width apart, heels straight, tops of feet pressing into the ground. Keep your elbows in close. Place your hands under your shoulders (see figure 10.10). Inhale and lift the upper spine, keeping your elbows slightly bent and tucked in toward the rib cage. Your hips should stay on the floor. Keep your shoulders down away from your ears and your chest open. Lengthen the crown of your head toward the sky and don't strain to tilt it back. Slide your tailbone toward your heels (see figure 10.11). Hold this pose for 5 to 10 deep breaths.

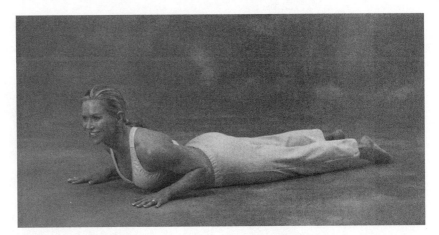

10.10 • Starting position

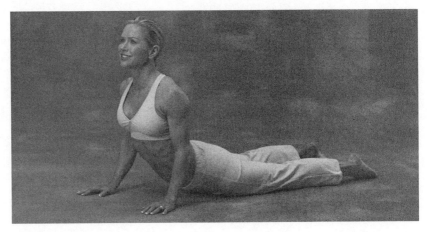

10.11 • Cobra

Reverse Tabletop

Start in a seated position with your legs bent. Keep your feet hip-width apart. Place your hands behind your body, fingertips facing forward, and inhale (see figure 10.12). Exhale and lift your hips toward the sky, pressing your weight into the heels of your feet and palms of your hands (see figure 10.13). Depending on the flexibility of your neck, gently release your head back and keep lifting your hips. Keep the navel pulled in toward the spine. Focus on opening your shoulders and chest. Keep your knees over your ankles and your hands underneath your shoulders. Stay here for 4 to 6 deep breaths.

This pose strengthens the wrists, shoulders, hips, thighs, and ankles. It increases the flexibility in the neck and tones the spine.

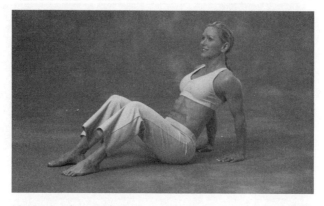

10.12 • Starting position

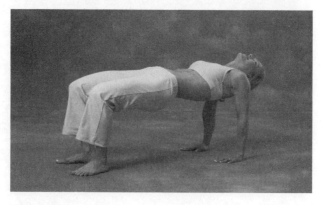

10.13 • Reverse Tabletop

Butterfly

Begin in a seated position with the soles of your feet together. If this is at all uncomfortable, place towels or small pillows under your knees. Put your hands on your ankles and press your elbows into your inside thighs. Gently push your knees toward the ground. Keep the sitting bones down toward the floor and lengthen the spine, allowing the crown of your head to reach up toward the sky. Drop the shoulders away from your ears and gently tuck your chin in (see figure 10.14). Inhale and exhale a little further into the stretch. Hold for 4 to 6 breaths.

The Butterfly improves the mobility and flexibility of the groin, hip, knee, and ankles.

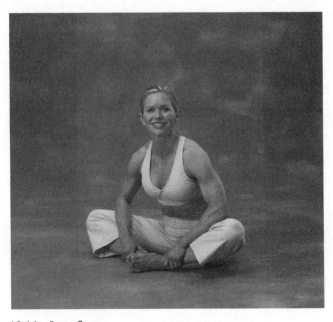

10.14 • Butterfly pose

Triangle

Step to the side with your right foot approximately three feet from your left. Point your right toes 90 degrees to the right. Move the toes of your left foot slightly to the right so that the foot is gently angled inward. Extend your arms straight out, parallel to the floor, with your shoulder blades relaxed. Imagine that your body is pressed against a pane of glass (see figure 10.15). Keep your hips stacked on top of each other as you tip over to the right, extending your left arm to the sky. Rest your right arm as far down your right leg as is comfortable. Keep your chest open and look toward the sky (see figure 10.16). (If this hurts your neck, turn your head toward the floor). Hold for 4 to 6 breaths and repeat on the other side.

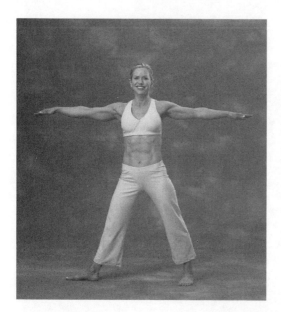

10.15 • Starting position

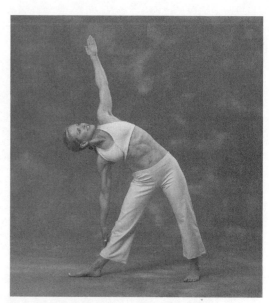

10.16 • Triangle pose

Relaxation Poses

Savasana/Corpse Pose

This asana is always practiced at the end of a yoga session. Cover your body with a blanket or put on a sweatshirt to keep yourself warm. The body cools off quickly after a yoga session and it's important to stay warm for this pose. If you suffer from lower back pain, place a pillow underneath your knees.

Start by lying on your back, extending your arms out to your sides, palms facing the sky. Extend your legs, let your feet fall open, and relax your hips (see figure 10.17). Relax the lower jaw and eyelids. Just melt into your mat. Allow your whole body to relax. Close your eyes and keep your breath relaxed and free of tension. Imagine your mind is like a wave in the water and let all of your thoughts just flow right past you. Imagine that a warm, dark feeling begins at the top of your forehead and flows all the way down to your toes. Continue to breathe comfortably, without effort. Feel the energy flow throughout your body, allowing your mind, body, and spirit to relax. Stay in this pose for five to ten minutes.

This pose helps to restore and replenish energy. When the mind is constantly bombarded with stimuli, it becomes overloaded. Savasana centers the mind and calms the body to help relieve insomnia, depression, lack of energy, and many other stress-related disorders.

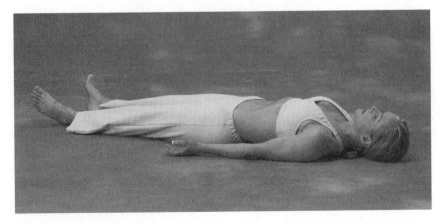

10.17 • Corpse pose

Easy Seated Pose

Sit in a cross-legged position with your ankles one in front of the other or one on top of the other. Relax your hands on your knees. Straighten your spine, gently tuck your chin in, and close your eyes. Allow your knees and hips to relax to either side (see figure 10.18). Feel your sitting bones rooted to the floor and the crown of your head lifting toward the sky. Soften your face, neck, and shoulders. Focus on the breath and try to let go of distractions. Hold this pose for 20 to 30 deep breaths.

This pose strengthens the mind and the body, calms the central nervous system, and invigorates the spirit. It helps to clear the mind of thoughts, strengthens the spine, and improves posture. Use it any time to bring the mind into the present and let go of past and future stresses.

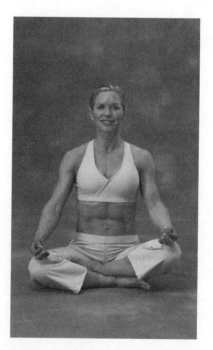

10.18 • Easy seated pose

Mountain Pose

Stand with your feet comfortably hip-width apart and distribute your weight evenly on both feet. Tighten your thigh muscles. Keep your pelvis in a neutral position, engaging your abdominals to avoid arching your back. Roll the shoulders up, back, and down, opening the heart center. Press all four corners of the feet down into the floor as the crown of your head lifts toward the sky, lengthening all your vertebrae. Drop the rib cage down, arms at your sides, fingers fanned to generate energy (see figure 10.19). Remain here for 10 deep breaths.

The Mountain pose helps to strengthen the posture, straighten the spine, and improve the alignment of the body.

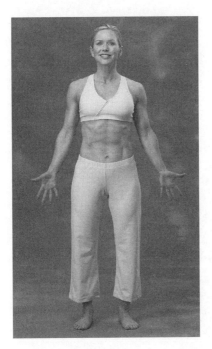

10.19 • Mountain pose

Child's Pose

Kneel and sit your hips back into your heels. Lower your upper body down over your lap and rest your forehead on the floor. Rest your arms at your sides, palms facing up (see figure 10.20). Or you can extend your arms overhead, reaching and spreading your fingers (see figure 10.21). Relax your neck, face, and shoulders. Take 5 to 10 deep, slow breaths.

This pose is relaxing *and* rejuvenating. It relieves tension in the neck, shoulders, and thoracic spine.

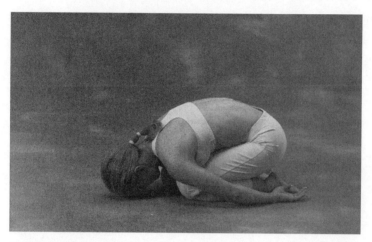

10.20 • Child's pose

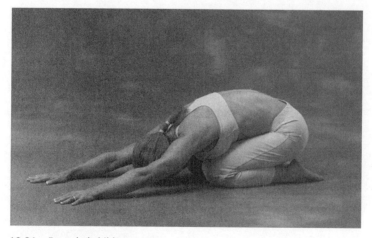

10.21 • Extended child's pose

After-Workout Stretches

Stretching after a workout is important because your muscles have constantly shortened from the repeated contractions of activity. Exercise also warms the muscles, so afterward is the best time to stretch and lengthen them. If you skip stretching to save time, you will gradually notice a decrease in flexibility and an increase in little aches and pains.

Let your body, your mood, and your schedule decide whether to do these stretches or the yoga workout. Yoga is best for overall flexibility and relaxation. The after-workout stretches are best after athletic activity.

Runner's Stretch

Stand in a lunge position, keeping your front knee above the ankle and balancing on your back toe (or you can drop your knee to the ground to modify). Press your open hip gently into the floor, lengthening the hip flexor muscles (see figure 10.22). Hold for 15 to 30 seconds and repeat on the other side.

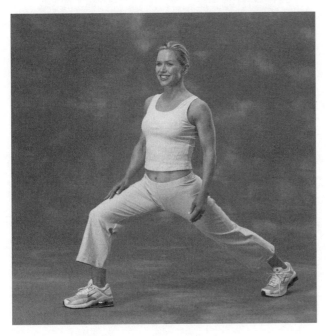

10.22 • Runner's stretch

Quadriceps Stretch

Stand up tall, balancing on one foot, or hold onto something nearby for support. Slowly bend one leg back and grasp the ankle or foot with the same-side hand. Keep the knee pointing down and close to the other leg. Keep breathing! Gently press your hips forward and draw the heel of the bent leg to your glutes (see figure 10.23). Hold for 15 to 30 seconds and repeat on the other side.

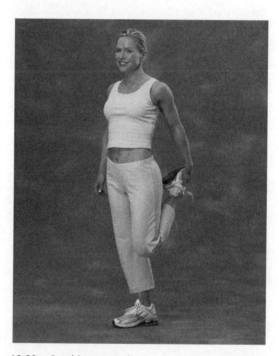

10.23 • Quadriceps stretch

Glutes Stretch

Lie on your back with both knees bent and feet flat on the floor. Lift your left leg, bend it, and rest your ankle against your right thigh. Gently grasp your hands underneath your right knee and pull your leg off the floor toward you. Keep your tailbone on the mat and feel the stretch through the buns and hips (see figure 10.24). Hold for 15 to 30 seconds and repeat on the other side.

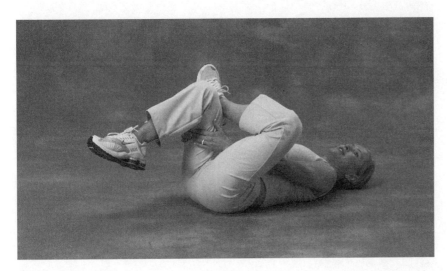

10.24 • Glutes stretch

Seated Hamstring Stretch

Sit tall on the floor with both legs extended in front of you. Slightly soften, or bend, the knees if your hamstrings are too tight. Keeping your back lengthened and your head neutral, take a deep breath and, as you exhale, slowly lean forward bending at the hip and coming over your legs (see figure 10.25).

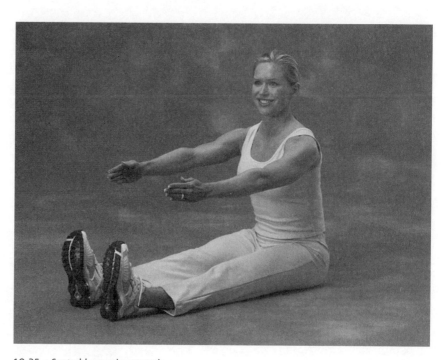

10.25 • Seated hamstring stretch

Calf Stretch

Standing with feet hip-width apart, bend your knees, dropping your glutes toward the floor. With fingertips on the floor for balance, dig your heels toward the floor, stretching the calves at the same time. Hold for 15 to 30 seconds (see figure 10.26).

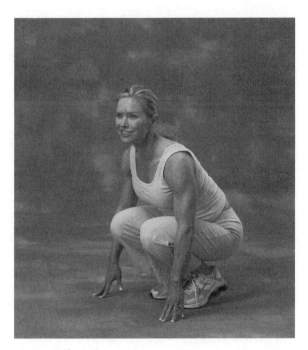

10.26 • Calf stretch

Shoulder Stretch

Bring one arm across the front of your chest with your elbow slightly bent. With the other hand, gently hold the elbow and pull the arm closer in toward the body. Hold for 15 to 30 seconds and repeat on the other side (see figure 10.27).

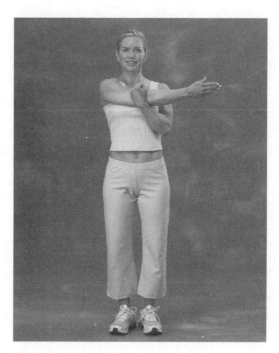

10.27 • Shoulder stretch

Tricep Stretch

Raise one arm straight overhead, bending at the elbow so your hand drops behind your head. With the other hand, gently grasp the bent elbow and slightly pull it farther behind your back. Keep the bent elbow near the ear (see figure 10.28). Hold for 15 to 30 seconds and repeat on the other side.

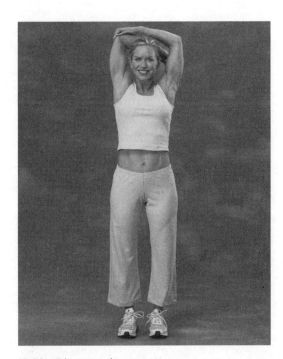

10.28 • Tricep stretch

Chest Stretch

Stand by a wall or doorway and raise your arm to shoulder height. Bending the elbow to 90 degrees with your fingers pointing up, press your hand and forearm against the wall or doorway. Lean the rest of your body gently forward until you feel a comfortable stretch in your chest (see figure 10.29). Hold for 15 to 30 seconds and repeat on the other side.

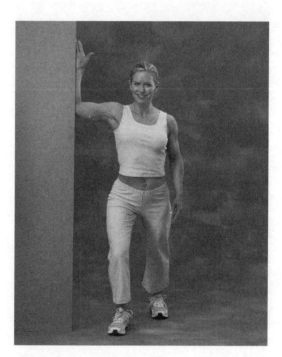

10.29 • Chest stretch

Torso Twist/Spinal Rotation

Lie on your back with knees bent at a 90-degree angle and your arms out to your sides (see figure 10.30). Keeping your shoulders relaxed and on the floor, inhale. As you exhale, drop both knees to one side (see figure 10.31). Hold for 2 or 3 seconds. Inhale again, slowly lifting your legs, and switch sides.

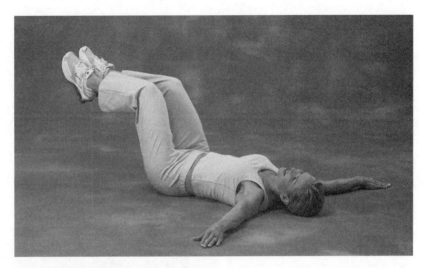

10.30 • Starting position

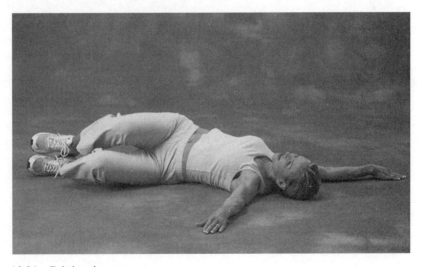

10.31 • Twisting the torso

Neck Stretch

Stand tall with your feet shoulder-width apart. Lengthening your shoulders away from your ears, gently tilt your head to the side, drawing your ear toward your shoulder. Hold for 2 to 3 seconds (see figure 10.32). Repeat on the other side.

Quick Tips

- Stretch after your body is properly warmed up and your body temperature is elevated.
- Move slowly.
- Try to increase your range of motion as you exhale. Inhale to prepare and exhale to sink further into a stretch.
- Don't overstretch. Never stretch to the point of pain.
- Pay attention to form and which muscle group you are stretching.

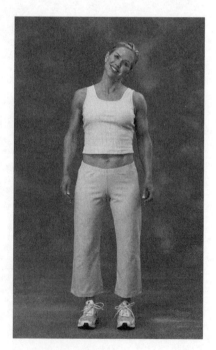

10.32 • Neck stretch

11 The Realistic Regimen:
A Healthy Plan for Putting It All Together

Now that you have the motivation to change your body for good, the knowledge you need about how your body works, and the tools you need to get the job done, you're ready to get started. Remember to begin at your pace—if you've been sedentary and you're carrying a few extra pounds, your muscles and joints will need time to adjust. Stick to this safe, moderate workout schedule for at least thirty days.

Remember—it takes sixty days to create a habit. So once you get to the end of Week 4, keep on going. Listen to your body. As you get stronger and healthier, challenge yourself gradually with heavier weights, longer distances, and different routines.

If you can't maintain this schedule at first, just do as much as you can do. If you can't do thirty minutes, start with ten. As long as you are consistent, you will get fitter and stronger. Try each day to go a little longer. And be patient with yourself!

Week One

DAY	CARDIO	STRENGTH	CORE	FLEX
Monday	30 minutes[1] (see chapter 7)			10 minutes Yoga[2] (see chapter 10)
Tuesday		20 minutes (see chapter 8—pick one upper body workout and one lower body workout[3])	10 minutes Pilates (see chapter 9)	
Wednesday	30 minutes[1] (see chapter 7)			10 minutes Yoga[2] (see chapter 10)
Thursday				
Friday	30 minutes[1] (see chapter 7)			10 minutes Yoga[2] (see chapter 10)
Saturday	Bonus day! Do 30 minutes[1] for extra credit! (see chapter 7)		10 minutes Pilates (see chapter 9)	
Sunday				

[1] If you can't do thirty full minutes, start at your level and do as much as you can. Five minutes is better than nothing!
[2] You can choose the ten after-workout stretches instead of yoga on any day.
[3] You can divide this workout into two days instead of one.

Week Two

DAY	CARDIO	STRENGTH	CORE	FLEX
Monday	30 minutes[1] (see chapter 7)			10 minutes Yoga[2] (see chapter 10)
Tuesday		20 minutes (see chapter 8—pick one upper body workout and one lower body workout[3])	10 minutes Pilates (see chapter 9)	
Wednesday	30 minutes[1] (see chapter 7)			10 minutes Yoga[2] (see chapter 10)
Thursday		20 minutes (see chapter 8—pick one upper body workout and one lower body workout[3])		
Friday	30 minutes[1] (see chapter 7)			10 minutes Yoga[2] (see chapter 10)
Saturday	Bonus day! Do 30 minutes[1] for extra credit! (see chapter 7)		10 minutes Pilates (see chapter 9)	
Sunday				

[1] If you can't do thirty full minutes, do as much as you can.
[2] You can choose the ten after-workout stretches instead of yoga on any day.
[3] You can divide this workout into two days instead of one.

Weeks Three and Four

DAY	CARDIO	STRENGTH	CORE	FLEX
Monday	30 minutes[1] (see chapter 7)			10 minutes Yoga[2] (see chapter 10)
Tuesday		20 minutes (see chapter 8—pick one upper body workout and one lower body workout[3])	10 minutes Pilates (see chapter 9)	
Wednesday	30 minutes[1] (see chapter 7)			10 minutes Yoga[2] (see chapter 10)
Thursday		20 minutes (see chapter 8—pick one upper body workout and one lower body workout[3])	10 minutes Pilates (see chapter 9)	
Friday	30 minutes[1] (see chapter 7)			10 minutes Yoga[2] (see chapter 10)
Saturday	30 minutes[1] (see chapter 7)	20 minutes (see chapter 8—pick one upper body workout and one lower body workout[3])		10 minutes Yoga[2] (see chapter 10)
Sunday	Do something active!			

WEEK 3   Add a little weight to each strength exercise.

WEEK 4   Add one extra set for each strength exercise.

[1] If you can't do thirty full minutes, do as much as you can.
[2] You can choose the ten after-workout stretches instead of yoga on any day.
[3] You can divide this workout into two days instead of one.

A WORKOUT LOG WORKS WONDERS

Want to make sure you really stick to your fitness plan? Put it in writing! Keeping a written workout log reinforces your commitment, giving you a real psychological edge. You'll get a powerful, satisfying feeling of accomplishment as you record your daily progress toward your health and fitness goals. Use the format outlined below or create your own. You can use a notebook or a three-ring binder or just create a document on your computer. You can download the following workout log from my website at www.motivatingbodies.com.

Daily Activity/Workout Log

Date:

Warm-up Activity

Spend five minutes moving your body gently, maybe even mimicking the movement you're going to do. If you're walking, walk slowly. If you're biking, bike slowly. Record your activity and the duration here.

Aerobic Exercise

Strengthen your heart and burn calories with the cardio machines or activities of your choice. Record your aerobic activities here.

Cardio exercise performed or equipment used. For example: "walk outdoors" or "walk on treadmill"	Level of resistance on cardio machine (if using)	Speed	Distance	Duration

Cool-Down Activity

Spend five minutes moving your body at a gentle pace. If you've been walking, walk slowly. If you've been biking, bike slowly. Record your activity and the duration here.

Strength Training

Build your muscles and boost your metabolism. Record your strength training activities here.

Exercise	Hand Weight or Resistance Band	Number of Reps	Number of Sets

Core Training

Whittle your middle and turn your torso into a powerhouse. Record your core workouts here.

Exercise	Number of Reps	Number of Sets

Flexibility Training

Choose the yoga pose workout or, if you're pressed for time, the after-workout stretches at the end of chapter 10. Record your poses or stretches here.

Yoga Poses	Stretches

Daily Thoughts

How did you do? How do you feel about it? Did you push too hard or not hard enough? Did you try something new? Give your mental muscles a workout and put your feelings into words here.

_____

_____

_____

Keeping a journal is important. If you choose not to use the daily log, if it takes too much time and effort, try using a small calendar instead. I recommend this for my busy personal training clients; I call it the "fitness map." We mark down each day we exercised, how much exercise we did, and whether we ate right. Keep the calendar handy—in the kitchen, in your briefcase, wherever it's most convenient. With a quick glance each week and each month, you can see how faithful you've been to your goals. Most of us can't rely on memory alone. I can barely remember what I did yesterday much less over the course of a month. You might be surprised to look back on a month you thought you did pretty well, only to see that, according to your calendar, you only managed to exercise twice a week!

EVERY JOURNEY NEEDS A MAP

The workouts in the previous chapters create a road map for a thirty-day journey. Each week we'll review and readjust our course. We'll steer clear of "road hazards" and "distractions" and stay focused on the road just like we have to do when we're behind the wheel. If you take your eyes off the road, you run the risk of getting into an accident.

And we'll deal with any bumps and ditches as we come to them. There will be times when your regimen goes off course. You'll catch a cold, pull a muscle, or get overwhelmed by a demanding project at work. I call these parking spots. They're just places where we stop for a bit. We don't stay there. When you hit a parking spot, just tell yourself you'll learn from it and avoid it in the future!

To avoid those parking spots, pull out your journal periodically and review the goals you set for yourself back in chapter 1. Make sure that each goal passes the S.M.A.R.T. test:

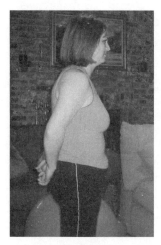
11.1 • Misti (before)

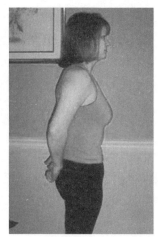
11.2 • Misti (after)

My television show, *Get Fit*, on ShopNBC puts me into the living rooms—and lives—of people around the country. I was thrilled to hear from one of my viewers, Misti T., who sent the story of her transformation along with the above photos.

Chris, I just wanted to thank you for all of your motivation in helping my girls and me get fit and healthy.

I am thirty-five and needed to lose fifteen pounds. So far, I have lost twelve with only three more to go. But most important is the health of my girls. I have an eight-year-old and a 4½-year-old and they could not be any different. My older daughter has asthma and after years on steroids is a bit "chunky." She always eats well and exercises but couldn't keep the weight off. My younger daughter is underweight with a condition known as bladder reflux and never eats. They both do the videos with me and we have started pretending that I am you and they are the models. It's so much fun to be exercising together!

My mom is the one who actually turned me on to you. She has been using your videos for a long time and also has such a motivating story. She suffered a major heart attack three years ago. Due to the grace of God and the wonderful surgeons, she survived and is better than ever! She loves your videos because of the ten-minute intervals and low impact. She recently had a medical checkup and learned that she had lost ten pounds that she didn't even realize she had lost! She has always been small but now she is buff! She had been trying to get me to use your videos for a long time, but I just wasn't into it. Then she said she "accidentally" ordered an extra workout video and wanted to know if I wanted to try it out. So I tried it on January 23, 2004, and have not missed a single day since! We even ordered the second tape and love to mix them up.

I am a registered nurse and work nights in the ER trauma center. Since I started with the plan I have so much more energy.

Thanks for making such a difference in our lives!

Specific: What kind of exercise am I doing? When am I doing it?

Measurable: How many minutes? What's my target heart rate?

Attainable: Is my body up to these challenges?

Realistic: Have I created a schedule I can stick to?

Time frame: What do I do each week? Each month?

Revisiting your goals every so often will help you to respond to the frustrations and temptations that can derail your commitment and send you backsliding into your old, bad habits. And it will remind you to adjust your program as your fitness level improves.

PARTING ADVICE FOR THE JOURNEY AHEAD

You now have the tools to continue on a lifelong journey to better health and fitness. They key to your success is in your hands, so put this book down and get moving! Your attitude will determine your success—stay positive and stay consistent. As I frequently tell my clients and viewers, there are no excuses for not moving at least ten minutes a day. Start with small changes to your diet and lifestyle, and think big. Your future belongs to you. I wish you great success on the road to better health!

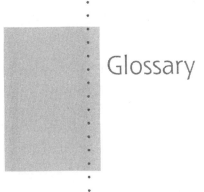

Glossary

Work and play are words used to describe the same thing under different conditions.

—MARK TWAIN

The world of health and fitness has a language all its own and some of the terms used by experts are abbreviations or nicknames, which may be tough to find in a typical dictionary. Here are some of the terms you may encounter.

Abs. Short for abdominals. A nickname used to describe the muscles of the abdomen. See chapter 9 for a complete description of these muscles.

Bicep. The muscle at the front of the upper arm. It's what you flex when you "make a muscle."

Carbs. Short for carbohydrates, your body's most accessible energy supply. They come in two varieties: simple carbohydrates, which are sugars, and complex carbohydrates. Carbohydrates are broken down into sugars in your small intestine so that they can be used to fuel your muscles, nerves, and brain.

Cardio. An abbreviation for the term "cardiovascular," used to refer to exercise that benefits the heart and circulatory system. Cardio exercises—like brisk walking, biking, and swimming—get your heart pumping and your blood moving.

Cholesterol. A fat found in our body tissues and those of other animals. There are two different kinds of cholesterol: HDL and LDL. HDL (high-density lipoprotein) cholesterol is good cholesterol. It actually helps rid your body of LDL (low-density lipoprotein), the bad cholesterol. High levels of LDL cholesterol in the blood are known to cause diseases of the heart and circulatory system.

Core. Also known as the "powerhouse." This term refers to the musculature of your midsection: front, back, and sides. Workouts (like the Pilates system) that target these muscles can flatten your tummy, narrow your waist, lengthen your posture, and strengthen your back.

Delt. A nickname for the deltoid, a shoulder muscle.

Dumbbells. The terms "dumbbells" and "hand weights" are used interchangeably, although "dumbbell" refers specifically to weights that are shaped like a rod with a disk at either end.

Flexion. This is a fancy term that means bending; it's the opposite of "extension."

Flies. Exercises that are done with the arms extended, so called because the motion resembles the movement of wings.

Free weights. These are weights, like dumbbells and barbells, that are not attached to a machine.

Glutes. Fitness professionals use this nickname to refer to the gluteus muscles, the large muscles of the buttocks.

Hamstrings. The tendons behind the knee.

Lats. The *latissimus dorsi* muscles, which are located in your midback.

Metabolism. The chemical processes by which your body obtains and uses energy and nutrients to sustain life.

Monounsaturated fat. Relatively healthy fats from vegetable sources like olive oil, canola oil, nuts, and avocados. Monounsaturated fats are thought to help lower your total blood cholesterol level. These are the healthiest fats.

Net carbs. Also known as "impact carbs." This is a new way of labeling the carbohydrate content of foods. The net carbs equal the total carbohydrates, in grams, minus the carbohydrates that have a minimal impact on blood sugar. For example: an energy bar nutrition label might indicate that the product has 20 grams of carbohydrates. Of these, 7 grams are fiber and 5 are from sugar alcohols. A "net carbs" calculation would subtract these from the total : 20 grams − 7 − 5 = 8 grams. This implies that only 8 grams of carbs would actually impact your blood sugar. Remember: The bottom line is that calories are calories!

Pilates. A system of strengthening and stretching exercises developed by Joseph Pilates in the early 1900s.

Polyunsaturated fats. Healthy (in moderation) fats found in nontropical plant oils like corn or soybean. These fats are thought to lower both good (HDL) and bad (LDL) cholesterol levels.

Quadriceps. The large muscle at the front of your thighs.

Rate of perceived exertion (RPE). A way of measuring, on a scale of one to ten, the amount of effort you feel as you're exercising.

Reps. Short for "repetitions," this term refers to the number of times you should perform an exercise.

Resistance training / strength training / weight training. These three terms are often used interchangeably to refer to exercise that builds muscle. Resistance training refers to building muscle by exerting it against resistance, such as resistance bands or the body's own weight (as in push-ups).

Weight training uses the resistance of weights to exert the muscle. Strength training refers to either kind of exercise.

Resting metabolic rate (RMR). The number of calories you need at rest to maintain all of your body's processes and systems such as digestion, breathing, circulation, tissue repair, and organ function.

Saturated fat. A kind of fat found in animal products that is associated with heart and circulatory problems.

Sets. Often used in strength training, this term refers to a group of repetitions—say, 10, 12, 15, or 20—you perform to exert a muscle to fatigue. Trainers will often tell you to do two or three sets of a particular exercise and rest thirty seconds to a minute between sets.

Trans fat. A chemically modified fat used by food manufacturers to prolong shelf life and provide a pleasant texture. These fats are even less healthy than saturated fats.

Triceps. The muscle located at the back of your upper arms.

Unsaturated fats. This term applies to both monounsaturated fats and polyunsaturated fats; both kinds of fats are derived from vegetable sources and both are healthy in small amounts.

Index